2ND Edition

BEST TENT
Camping

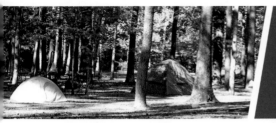

ILLINOIS

YOUR CAR-CAMPING GUIDE TO SCENIC BEAUTY, THE SOUNDS
OF NATURE, AND AN ESCAPE FROM CIVILIZATION

Best Tent Camping: Illinois

Published by Menasha Ridge Press
Distributed by Publishers Group West
Printed in the United States of America
Second edition, first printing

Library of Congress Cataloging-in-Publication Data

Names: Schirle, John, author.
Title: Best tent camping, Illinois : your car-camping guide to scenic beauty, the sounds of nature, and an escape from
   civilization / John Schirle.
Other titles: Best in tent camping, Illinois
Description: Second Edition. | Birmingham, Alabama : Menasha Ridge Press, an imprint of AdventureKEEN, [2018] |
   "Distributed by Publishers Group West"—T.p. verso. | Includes index.
Identifiers: LCCN 2018018932| ISBN 9781634041041 (paperback) | ISBN 9781634041058 (ebook)
Subjects: LCSH: Camping—Illinois—Guidebooks. | Camp sites, facilities, etc.—Illinois—Guidebooks. |
   Outdoor recreation—Illinois—Guidebooks. | Illinois—Guidebooks.
Classification: LCC GV191.42.I3 S33 2018 | DDC 796.5409773—dc23
LC record available at https://lccn.loc.gov/2018018932

Cover and book design: Jonathan Norberg
Maps: Thomas Hertzel, Steve Jones, and John Schirle
Interior photos: John Schirle unless otherwise noted
Indexing: Rich Carlson

 MENASHA RIDGE PRESS
An imprint of AdventureKEEN
2204 First Ave. S., Ste. 102
Birmingham, AL 35233
800-443-7227, fax 205-326-1012

Visit menasharidge.com for a complete listing of our books and for ordering information. Contact us at our website, at
facebook.com/menasharidge, or at twitter.com/menasharidge with questions or comments. To find out more about
who we are and what we're doing, visit blog.menasharidge.com.

Front cover: Main photo: Camel Rock at Garden of the Gods Recreation Area (see page 134)
   by Jeffery Alan Brown/Shutterstock.com
Inset photo: Pine Hills Campground (see page 149) by John M. Hagstrom/Flickr.com

2ND Edition

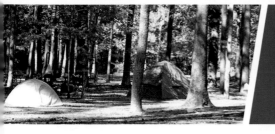

BEST ⛺ TENT
Camping

ILLINOIS

YOUR CAR-CAMPING GUIDE TO SCENIC BEAUTY, THE SOUNDS
OF NATURE, AND AN ESCAPE FROM CIVILIZATION

John Schirle

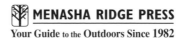

MENASHA RIDGE PRESS
Your Guide to the Outdoors Since 1982

Illinois Campground Locator Map

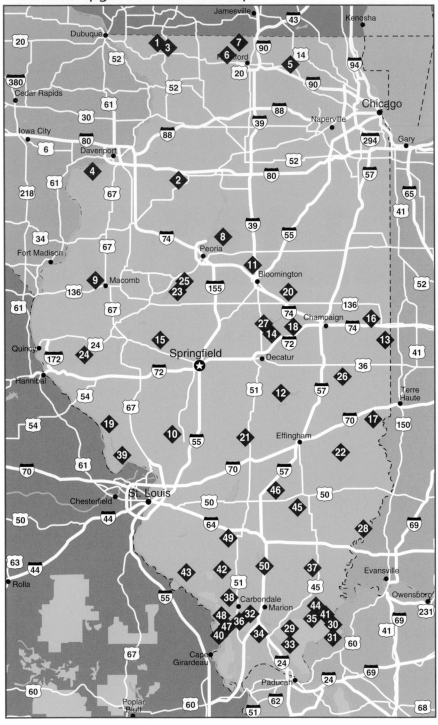

CONTENTS

SOUTHERN ILLINOIS   110

Map Legend

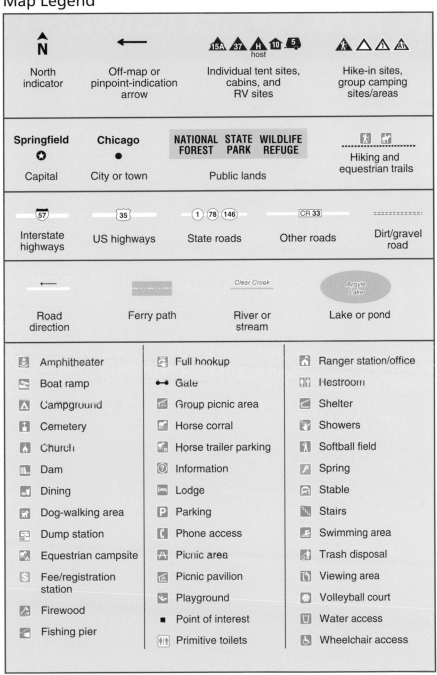

North indicator

Off-map or pinpoint-indication arrow

Individual tent sites, cabins, and RV sites

Hike-in sites, group camping sites/areas

Springfield — **Capital**

Chicago — **City or town**

NATIONAL FOREST / STATE PARK / WILDLIFE REFUGE — **Public lands**

Hiking and equestrian trails

Interstate highways

US highways

State roads

Other roads

Dirt/gravel road

Road direction

Ferry path

River or stream

Lake or pond

Amphitheater	Full hookup	Ranger station/office
Boat ramp	Gate	Restroom
Campground	Group picnic area	Shelter
Cemetery	Horse corral	Showers
Church	Horse trailer parking	Softball field
Dam	Information	Spring
Dining	Lodge	Stable
Dog-walking area	Parking	Stairs
Dump station	Phone access	Swimming area
Equestrian campsite	Picnic area	Trash disposal
Fee/registration station	Picnic pavilion	Viewing area
Firewood	Playground	Volleyball court
Fishing pier	Point of interest	Water access
	Primitive toilets	Wheelchair access

ACKNOWLEDGMENTS

A huge thanks to all the personnel at the Illinois Department of Natural Resources, the U.S. Forest Service, the U.S. Fish & Wildlife Service, and the various county conservation districts and forest preserves across Illinois that provided so much help as I researched this book. They patiently answered my questions, responded to my phone calls and emails, and even gave me guided tours around their properties. Illinois has tremendous natural beauty, but it is carefully maintained and kept accessible only through the often-unsung efforts of these folks.

Thanks to all the readers of the first edition, and for their many encouraging and helpful emails and reviews.

Thanks to Mary Handley, who taught me at Stephen Decatur High School to delight in writing.

Thanks to my coworkers at the Decatur Public Library Children's Department, who graciously juggled schedules to allow me time to travel and camp.

Thanks to my good friend Mark Sturgell, who not only encouraged me along the way but also painstakingly proofread every campground profile in the first edition, helping me see what I had missed.

Thanks to the folks at Menasha Ridge Press, who patiently worked with this first-time author to create what I hope is a helpful addition to an excellent series.

Thanks above all to God, who crafted the prairies, forests, canyons, bluffs, rivers, and lakes that are Illinois today and gave them to us to care for and enjoy.

—John Schirle

PREFACE

If you've picked up this book, I expect that camping for you, like me, is not just overnight lodging—it's part of the entire outdoor experience. You want to pitch your tent on soft grass surrounded by woods, to be lulled to sleep by the sound of a nearby creek, to wake to watch the sunrise across the lake. (Just reading these words probably makes you want to pull out your calendar to find your next free weekend.) For years I've searched the Midwest for such perfect spots, and found that websites and even most books don't tell the whole story. That's why I was delighted to stumble across Menasha Ridge Press's *Best Tent Camping: Missouri and the Ozarks*, which accompanied me on several wonderful trips. I was even more delighted when Menasha Ridge asked if I'd be willing to author this volume on my home state of Illinois.

Exploring Illinois for this book has been fun. From north to south and from east to west, it's been an adventure, discovering so many wonderful rivers to canoe, lakes to fish, trails to hike, woods to wander, and quiet places to camp. I knew some places I wanted to include from the start (like my all-time favorite, Ferne Clyffe State Park), but as I traversed the state, first by phone and Internet and then by car, I uncovered more and more fascinating and diverse wild places that I had to share. Some were places I'd long wanted to visit, such as Apple River Canyon State Park to the northwest, with its bubbling creeks and steep ravines. Others were completely off my radar, surprises that I stumbled upon, such as the virtually unvisited McCully Heritage Project to the southwest or Lodge Park along the Sangamon River, barely 30 miles from my hometown. I kept discovering new places—the research was so much fun that the hardest part was to stop exploring and start writing!

Knowing that "ideal campsite" conjures different images for each of us, I've tried to include a variety of campgrounds. All have nonelectric sites in a natural setting, and most either don't attract RVs or have separate RV and tent areas. Some have few or no amenities but offer secluded sites where you're almost sure to be by yourself. Others offer a shower building, restaurant, and store. At some you can fish, hike, boat, bike, swim, or even go rock-climbing; others are perfect for simply relaxing. Many are near other natural or historic sites, so I've also included descriptions of those. Among them, I hope you will find places that are a perfect fit.

Since the publication of the first edition, I've continued to camp and explore Illinois. I've received lots of feedback and suggestions from other campers through email, informal conversations, and programs where I've presented the book. In this edition you'll find some new campgrounds, replacing others that were no longer a best choice, and lots of new suggestions for places to explore in and around those that were in the first edition. I found that many details had changed since the first edition, and everything has been checked and updated.

I hope I've been thorough and doubt I've been exhaustive. I'm sure tucked away in some corner of the state—or perhaps just a few miles down the road—is yet another camping getaway, kept secret by the few who visit it year after year. If you encounter some special place that deserves to be included in a future edition of this book (and don't mind sharing the secret!), let me know at illinoiscamper@gmail.com.

Meanwhile, throw your gear in the car and head out to explore the Prairie State!

BEST CAMPGROUNDS

BEST FOR CANOEING

BEST FOR CYCLING/MOUNTAIN BIKING

BEST FOR FISHING

BEST FOR HIKING

BEST FOR HIKING *(continued)*

BEST FOR SWIMMING

BEST FOR FAMILIES WITH KIDS

BEST FOR BEAUTY

BEST FOR PRIVACY

BEST FOR SPACIOUSNESS

BEST FOR QUIET

BEST FOR SECURITY

BEST FOR CLEANLINESS

INTRODUCTION

HOW TO USE THIS GUIDEBOOK

Menasha Ridge Press welcomes you to *Best Tent Camping: Illinois.* Whether you are new to this activity or have been sleeping in your portable outdoor shelter over decades of outdoor adventures, please review the following information. It explains how we have worked with the author to organize this book and how you can make the best use of it.

THE RATINGS SYSTEM

As with all books in the Best Tent Camping series, the author personally experienced dozens of campgrounds and campsites to select the top 50 locations in this state. Within that universe of 50 sites, the author then ranked each one in the six categories described below. As a tough grader, the author awarded few five-star ratings, but each campground in this guidebook is superlative in its own way. For example, a site may be rated only one star in one category but perhaps five stars in another category. This rating system allows you to choose your destination based on the attributes that are most important to you.

★★★★★	The site is **ideal** in that category.
★★★★	The site is **exemplary** in that category.
★★★	The site is **very good** in that category.
★★	The site is **above average** in that category.
★	The site is **acceptable** in that category.

BEAUTY

Beauty, of course, is in the eye of the beholder, but panoramic views or proximity to a lake or river earn especially high marks. A campground that blends in well with the environment scores well, as do areas with remarkable wildlife or geology. Well-kept vegetation and nicely laid-out sites also up the ratings.

PRIVACY

The number of sites in a campground, the amount of screening between them, and physical distance from one another are decisive factors for the privacy ratings. Other considerations include the presence of nearby trails or day-use areas, and proximity to a town or city that would invite regular day-use traffic and perhaps compromise privacy.

SPACIOUSNESS

The size of the tent spot, its proximity to other tent spots, and whether or not it is defined or bordered from activity areas are the key considerations. The highest ratings go to sites that allow the tent camper to comfortably spread out without overlapping neighboring sites or picnic, cooking, or parking areas.

QUIET

Criteria for this rating include several touchstones: the author's experience at the site, the nearness of roads, the proximity of towns and cities, the probable number of RVs, the likelihood of noisy all-terrain vehicles or boats, and whether a campground host is available or willing to enforce the quiet hours. Of course, one set of noisy neighbors can deflate a five-star rating into a one-star (or no-star), so the latter criterion—campground enforcement—was particularly important in the author's evaluation in this category.

SECURITY

How you determine a campground's security will depend on what you view as the greater risk: other people or the wilderness. The more remote the campground, the less likely you are to run into opportunistic crime but the harder it is to get help in case of an accident or a dangerous wildlife confrontation. Ratings in this category take into consideration whether there is a campground host or resident park ranger, proximity of other campers' sites, how much day traffic the campground receives, how close the campground is to a town or city, and whether there is cell phone reception or some type of phone or emergency call button.

CLEANLINESS

A campground's appearance often depends on who was there right before you and how your visit coincides with the maintenance schedule. In general, higher marks have gone to those campgrounds with hosts who cleaned up regularly. The rare case of odor-free toilets also gleaned high marks. At unhosted campgrounds, criteria included trash receptacles and evidence that sites were cleared and that signs and buildings were kept repaired. Markdowns for the campground were not given for a single visitor's garbage left at a site, but old trash in the shrubbery and along trails, indicating infrequent cleaning, did secure low ratings.

THE CAMPGROUND PROFILE

Each profile contains a concise but informative narrative that describes the campground and individual sites. Readers get a sense not only of the property itself but also the recreational opportunities available nearby. This descriptive text is enhanced with three helpful sidebars: Ratings, Key Information, and Getting There (accurate driving directions that lead you to the campground from the nearest major roadway).

THE CAMPGROUND LOCATOR MAP AND MAP LEGEND

Use the Illinois Campground Locator Map, opposite the Table of Contents on page iv, to assess the exact location of each campground. The campground's number appears not only on the overview map but also in the table of contents and on the profile's first page.

A map legend that details the symbols found on the campground-layout maps appears immediately following the Table of Contents, on page vii.

CAMPGROUND-LAYOUT MAPS

Each profile contains a detailed map of campground sites, internal roads, facilities, and other key items.

GPS CAMPGROUND-ENTRANCE COORDINATES

All of the profiles in this guidebook include the GPS coordinates for each site entrance. The intersection of the latitude (north) and longitude (west) coordinates orient you at the entrance.

Please note that this guidebook uses the degree decimal-minute format for presenting the GPS coordinates. Example:

N42° 26.932'   W90° 03.033'

To convert GPS coordinates from degrees, minutes, and seconds to the above degree decimal-minute format, the seconds are divided by 60. For more on GPS technology, visit usgs.gov.

A note of caution: Actual GPS devices will easily guide you to any of these campgrounds, but users of smartphone mapping apps may find that cell phone service is sometimes unavailable in the remote areas where some of these hideaways are located.

WEATHER

Folks in Illinois often joke that if you don't like the weather, just wait an hour. Within each of the four seasons there can be a lot of variability, and conditions can change considerably even during a single day.

Spring varies between rainy and overcast to sunny and moderate. I have hiked in short sleeves on warm days in March, and I've also seen the rare snow or ice storm in April. Many parks with seasonal campgrounds and trails do not open them until late April or May because of muddy conditions. April–June is also Illinois's main tornado season.

Memorial Day is considered the unofficial start of summer recreation, but even into June the evenings can be cool enough to make flannel shirts and jackets welcome. July and particularly August are usually hot and humid, and you may encounter unexpected thunderstorms, even on an otherwise clear day.

Fall is my favorite season for camping, with more moderate temperatures and less humidity, but conditions can fluctuate. Daytime highs may be very comfortable (50s–70s) even as late as Thanksgiving, but cold at night. Other days will be wet, windy, and chilly. One year, when I camped in early October, on some nights it got to freezing and on other nights a long-sleeved shirt was sufficient.

Except around Lake Michigan, Illinois does not see a lot of snow most years in the winter, but it can get very cold. Equally important, ice and sleet can impact travel conditions, and even when roadways are clear, the trails, bike paths, and campgrounds may still be slippery.

A couple of experiences with unexpected storms have taught me to always camp with some way to access weather information. Smartphone weather apps are ideal, but in some rural areas service may be spotty or nonexistent. A weather radio with backup batteries is most reliable.

FIRST AID KIT

A useful first aid kit may contain more items than you might think necessary. These are just the basics. Prepackaged kits in waterproof bags are available. Even though quite a few items are listed here, they pack down into a small space.

- Adhesive bandages, such as Band-Aids

- Antibiotic ointment (Neosporin or the generic equivalent)

- Antiseptic or disinfectant, such as Betadine or hydrogen peroxide

- Benadryl or the generic equivalent, diphenhydramine (in case of allergic reactions)

- Butterfly-closure bandages

- Elastic bandages or joint wraps

- Emergency poncho

- Epinephrine in a prefilled syringe (for severe allergic reactions to bee stings, etc.)

- Gauze (one roll and six 4-by-4-inch pads)

- Ibuprofen or acetaminophen

- Insect repellent

- LED flashlight or headlamp

- Matches or pocket lighter

- Mirror for signaling passing aircraft

- Moleskin/Spenco 2nd Skin

- Pocketknife or multipurpose tool

- Sunscreen/lip balm

- Waterproof first aid tape

- Whistle (it's more effective in signaling rescuers than your voice)

FLORA AND FAUNA PRECAUTIONS

POISONOUS PLANTS

Poison oak and sumac are not common in Illinois, but poison ivy is widespread. Recognizing and avoiding contact with poison ivy is the most effective way to prevent the itchy rash this plant causes. In Illinois, poison ivy can be a small ground plant or climbing vine, with leaflets in clusters of three. The leaves vary in shape, but in Illinois the two outer leaves typically have a single large lobe on the outside edge and not the inside, looking like a mitten.

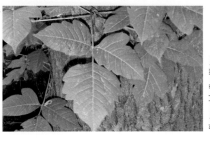

Photograph by Tom Watson

Urushiol, a type of oil in the plant, is responsible for the rash and may be present even in the dead or leafless vine. You can get the rash by direct contact with the plant or by later touching shoes, clothing, hiking gear, or even pets on which the oil has rubbed off. As soon after contact as possible, washing the affected skin with alcohol, soap, and water can prevent the rash from developing. If you know you get the rash easily (as I do), always wear long pants when hiking through underbrush and carry an alcohol-based hand sanitizer and a washcloth along with your drinking water. Be sure to eventually wash off shoes, gear, pets, and anything else that may have the oil on it.

If you are exposed to poison ivy, raised lines or blisters will usually appear within 12 hours (but sometimes much later), accompanied by a terrible itch. Refrain from scratching because it can cause infection, but it won't spread the rash, as is commonly believed. Wash and dry the area thoroughly. Various over-the-counter products will alleviate the symptoms until it heals on its own. In worse cases, a doctor can prescribe treatment.

EMERALD ASH BORER

The emerald ash borer (*Agrilus planipennis*) is an exotic insect, native to Asia, which currently threatens ash trees in the Great Lakes region. The pest has been found in much of Illinois and can be spread inadvertently in infested firewood. There is no longer an official ban against moving firewood within Illinois, but it is still discouraged, and some campgrounds may have specific rules against bringing in firewood from outside the area. By following some simple rules, you can help prevent the spread of these destructive insects.

- Purchase aged firewood near your campsite location; don't bring it from home. Many parks sell firewood, often delivered right to your site, and it is often available from vendors just outside the parks.

- Firewood purchased at or near your destination should be used during your camping trip; don't take it to another destination.

- Buy wood that has no bark or loose bark (a sign the wood is very dry). This will reduce the chances of infestation while also making your fire easier to start.

MOSQUITOES

Mosquitoes are common throughout Illinois. Although it's not a common occurrence, individuals can become infected with the West Nile virus by being bitten by an infected mosquito. Culex mosquitoes, the primary varieties that can transmit West Nile virus to humans, thrive in urban rather than natural areas. Most people infected with West Nile virus have no symptoms of illness, but some may become ill, usually 3–15 days after being bitten.

In Illinois, summer is the time thought to be the highest risk period for West Nile virus. At this time of the year—and any time you expect mosquitoes to be buzzing around—you may want to wear protective clothing, such as long sleeves, long pants, and socks. Loose-fitting, light-colored clothing is best. Spray your clothing with insect repellent. Follow the instructions on the repellent and take extra care with children.

RACCOONS

Most wooded areas in Illinois are home to at least some raccoons, which have learned to take advantage of the buffet of foodstuffs we regularly leave out for their enjoyment. I've seen industrious raccoons break into locked coolers and crawl through barely opened car windows to get to scraps of food. To avoid their nocturnal visits:

- Never have any food—not even candy, gum, soft drinks, or beer—in your tent.

- Promptly dispose of all garbage with any trace of food on it. If an enclosed trash container is not available, put the garbage sack in a closed vehicle for the night.

- Wipe up or pick up any spilled food.

If you've been cooking meat, raccoons' inquisitive noses may draw them to your camp-site, but if you've disposed of everything, let them sniff around and they'll soon determine there's nothing left and wander off.

SNAKES

The snakes you will most likely see while hiking in Illinois are nonvenomous. The best rule is to leave all snakes alone, give them a wide berth as you hike past, and make sure any hiking companions (including dogs) do the same.

There are four species of venomous snakes in Illinois: the copperhead, cottonmouth, timber rattlesnake *(see below)*, and massasauga. The first three are found only in the southernmost one-third to one-quarter of the state, while the endangered massasauga is found in scattered locations in just a few counties. In many years and miles of hiking Illinois trails, I have only seen live venomous snakes in one place: the LaRue–Pine Hills (see the Pine Hills Campground profile on page 149).

Venomous snakes are not aggressive and tend to bite people only when stepped on, picked up, or cornered. If you are entering an area where they might be (and I've noted some of these areas), take a few simple precautions. Wear over-the-ankle boots and loose-fitting long pants. Stay on established trails, do not step or put your hands beyond your range of detailed visibility, and avoid wandering around in the dark. Step onto logs and rocks, never over them (in case a snake might be sheltering on the other side). Always avoid walking through dense brush.

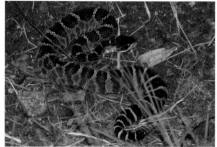

Photograph by Jane Huber

TICKS

Ticks like to hang out in the brush and the tall grass that grows around campsites and along trails. They're most numerous during hot summer months, but you should be tick-aware throughout the year. Two varieties are prevalent in Illinois: dog ticks and deer ticks. The latter are the primary carriers of Lyme disease, and may be so tiny that you'll have to look carefully to spot them. You may see them on shoes, socks, or hats, and they can take several hours to actually latch on. Both varieties may carry disease, but it requires several hours of actual attachment before it can be transmitted.

If you're going to hike where ticks are prevalent, the best prevention is to wear light-colored clothes (so you can see the ticks more readily), long pants tucked into your socks, closed shoes, and an insect repellent with DEET. Check yourself visually several times a day and your whole body carefully at least once a day. Ticks like to migrate to warm dark places like the back of the knee, inside the thighs, under the waistband or sock elastic, or in the belly button or armpit. Ticks that haven't attached are easily removed but not easily killed. If you pick off a tick in the woods, just toss it aside. If you find one on your body at camp, toss it into the toilet or the fire (otherwise it may find you again). For ticks that have attached themselves, it's best to remove them with tweezers. Grasp the tick behind the head as close to the skin surface as possible and pull straight back with a slow steady force, avoiding crushing the tick's body. Thoroughly disinfect the bite site. Practically all tick bites will result in some local redness and itching, but that doesn't mean you've contracted a disease.

STATE PARKS

About two-thirds of the campgrounds I've included are managed by the Illinois Department of Natural Resources (IDNR). These include any labeled state parks, state recreation areas, state forests, and state fish and wildlife areas. (And if you're not sure what category a particular spot is, don't worry, sometimes the IDNR isn't either—the road sign may say "state recreation area," while the official website calls it a "state fish and wildlife area," and the ranger will answer the phone with "state park.")

Though the IDNR fees listed are applicable to most campers, certain discounts are available for Illinois residents who are seniors, disabled, disabled veterans, or former POWs. Discounts vary depending on the day of the week and the class of campsite. Check bit.ly /IDNRCampingFees for details.

At many IDNR campgrounds, you can reserve some campsites, cabins, and shelters at least three days in advance via reserveamerica.com for a $5 nonrefundable fee per reservation. Search for the name of the park, then the type and location of the desired site. Where reservations are possible, it's usually for the Class A or B sites with electricity, since they are more in demand. Reservations are usually not accepted (or needed) for walk-in or primitive Class C or D sites.

Note that IDNR personnel wear many hats, and aren't always in the office or next to the phone. When calling or visiting a park office, if you don't find someone there or get an immediate response, leave a message and be patient. They'll get back to you as soon as possible.

SHAWNEE NATIONAL FOREST

The only national forest in Illinois, the Shawnee has more than 275,000 acres of woods and meadows, hills and canyons, and lakes, rivers, and streams. There is ample room for hiking, camping, backpacking, fishing, hunting, rock-climbing, or horseback riding. Six of the campgrounds in this book are on national forest land.

In addition, primitive camping is allowed on national forest land outside the boundaries of developed campgrounds and picnic areas. Camping is not allowed within designated natural areas, within research natural areas, within 150 feet of a municipal water source, or within a quarter-mile of a developed campground or picnic area. There is no fee for camping in general forest areas; however, a maximum of 14 days of continuous use applies. If you do camp outside a developed campground, be sure you follow all regulations and recommendations for fires and waste disposal. Check bit.ly/ShawneeDispersedCamping for detailed information.

CAMPGROUND ETIQUETTE

Here are some simple tips to keep you on good terms with your camping neighbors, campground personnel, and all of us who will come camping after you.

- **OBTAIN ALL PERMITS AND AUTHORIZATIONS REQUIRED.** Make sure you check in, pay your fee, and mark your site as directed. If the sign says to check in first, but you'd like to visually scope out the sites first, just ask.

- **FOLLOW THE CAMPGROUND'S RULES.** Observe rules regarding building fires, facility usage, parking, checkout times, number of people per site, etc.; ask if you need an exception. If the rule says six people per site but your nephew makes seven, check in advance if that would be acceptable. Most campground hosts are flexible with reasonable requests.

- **LEAVE ONLY FOOTPRINTS.** Be sensitive to the ground beneath you. Be sure to place all garbage in designated receptacles or pack it out if none are available. If there was trash when you arrived, take care of it as well, and leave the campsite better than you found it. Never burn trash—trash smoke smells and trash debris in a fire ring is unsightly.

- **PLAN AHEAD.** Know your equipment, your ability, and the area in which you are camping, and prepare accordingly. Be self-sufficient at all times; carry necessary supplies for changes in weather and other conditions.

- **BE COURTEOUS TO OTHER CAMPERS, HIKERS, BIKERS, AND OTHERS YOU ENCOUNTER.** Respect their privacy and space unless invited—don't hike through their site to get to yours. If there are other choices, don't set up camp next to someone who has obviously selected a secluded site. It may be the best area of the campground, but they got there first, so you should look elsewhere. Avoid, if you can, arriving late at night and attempting to set up camp in the glare of your headlights. If you must arrive late, look for a site away from others, plan to light a lantern, unload all at once (so you don't have to keep slamming car doors), and set up quietly. Keep the noise level down in your party, even if it's not officially quiet hours. If you camp with a dog, be sure it doesn't bark at passersby or at noises in the night. Keep it leashed and clean up after it. Dog waste is not the same as wild animal waste. Those camping after you won't want to deal with it, and it can be harmful to the environment.

HAPPY CAMPING

There is nothing worse than a bad camping trip, especially because it is so easy to have a great time. To assist with making your outing a happy one, here are some pointers:

- **DO SOME HOMEWORK.** Since you're reading this book, I expect that you, like me, prefer to research before traveling. I want to know all there is to see and do in the area: trails to hike, historic sites, museums, even restaurants. I may not choose to visit them all, but knowing the options helps me plan. Check the resources in Appendix B. Remember, though, that even official websites aren't always regularly updated.

- **RESERVE YOUR SITE IN ADVANCE** whenever possible If a campground is very popular or it's a prime weekend.

- **CALL AHEAD.** There are times you just throw the gear in the car and hit the road, but whenever possible call at least a week in advance. The details in this book were correct at publication, but fees go up, office hours change, and any number of unforeseen events can close campgrounds or limit services. Don't just ask: "Are you open?" Be specific. Confirm details that are important to you: "Is the beach open?" "How are the bass biting?" "What's the condition of the mountain hiking trail?" Ask if there are any local events that would attract a larger-than-usual crowd during your visit. Double-check driving directions— rural roads may temporarily close due to flooding or other circumstances.

- **PICK YOUR CAMPING BUDDIES WISELY.** Make sure you're all on the same page regarding expectations, sleeping arrangements, food requirements, and activity plans. If you want to hike while your friend would rather fish, that can work, as long as you've communicated in advance. If he wants showers and flush toilets but you plan to backpack, one of you may be disappointed. If camping with a group, select a campground that will make everyone comfortable. Many state park campgrounds offer primitive sites, RV sites, and air-conditioned cabins all within a short walk of each other.

- **JUST SAY "NO" TO HOLIDAYS.** Most campgrounds are busiest over Memorial Day, July Fourth, Labor Day, and sometimes even Columbus Day. Unless your annual family outing is on one of those weekends, avoid camping then. If you must, there are some campgrounds in the book where sites are so spread out (such as Trail of Tears State Forest) that you can still find relative seclusion. My preference is to camp midweek, when traffic is lighter. The only downside is that special programs (guided hikes, live music, historic building tours, hayrides, etc.) at some parks are often only scheduled for weekends, when more people are there to participate.

- **DRESS APPROPRIATELY FOR THE SEASON AND FOR YOUR ACTIVITIES.** It may be warm and sunny when you leave home but turn cold and wet by the time you bed down at your campsite. Bring extra clothes, wear layers of clothes, and plan for extremes. If you'll be hiking, bring appropriate, comfortable, and sturdy footwear.

- **PITCH YOUR TENT ON A LEVEL SURFACE,** preferably one covered with leaves, pine straw, or grass. If rain is possible, make sure the site is not lower than the surrounding area and prone to flooding. Do a little site maintenance first, such as picking up small rocks and sticks that can damage the tent and make sleeping uncomfortable. Pitch your tent on a tarp to keep out ground moisture and to protect the tent floor. Look up as well and check for standing dead or storm-damaged trees. These may have loose or broken limbs that can fall at any time.

- **TAKE A SLEEPING PAD** if you don't like sleeping on the ground. Get one that is full-length and thicker than you might think you need. You'll sleep more comfortably and warmly.

- **IF YOU TEND TO USE THE BATHROOM AT NIGHT, PLAN ACCORDINGLY.** Keep a flashlight, shoes, and whatever else you might need near the tent door, and know where you need to head in the dark.

- **PLAN FOR TASTY, FUN, AND EASY MEALS.** If you're not backpacking, there's no reason to skimp on food due to weight, so bring what you need. It's especially fun when camping with others to cook and eat around the campfire. With a little planning, you can prepackage and precook some ingredients to make great meals with easy preparation and cleanup. You can find plenty of books and websites with suggestions: I like trailcooking.com.

- **BRING A KID OR TWO.** I've taken lots of kids on camping, hiking, caving, canoeing, and fishing trips, and can testify that the outdoors seems all the more adventurous and wonderful when seen through the eyes of a fifth-grader spending his first night in a tent. Take your own kids, grandkids, nieces, or nephews, of course, but how about also inviting a couple of their friends, a coworker and his kids, or a friend and her daughter? The natural world can be transformational for kids, particularly in the modern era, when video games and texting are replacing old-fashioned outdoor play. Pick your campground and activities appropriate to the age, experience, and energy level (usually high) of the kids. I've included several spots with interesting hikes, swimming beaches, interactive exhibits, and even kid-friendly programs.

A WORD ABOUT BACKCOUNTRY CAMPING

Following these guidelines will increase your chances for a pleasant, safe, and low-impact interaction with nature.

- **ADHERE TO THE ADAGES "PACK IT IN, PACK IT OUT" AND "TAKE ONLY PICTURES, LEAVE ONLY FOOTPRINTS."** Practice Leave No Trace camping ethics while in the backcountry.

- **IN ILLINOIS, OPEN FIRES ARE PERMITTED** except during dry times when authorities may issue a fire ban. Consider bringing a lightweight backpacking stove instead, which is often easier and more reliable.

- **HANG FOOD AWAY FROM ANIMALS** to prevent them from becoming introduced to (and dependent on) human food. Wildlife learns to associate backpacks and backpackers with easy food sources, thereby influencing their behavior.

- **BURY SOLID HUMAN WASTE** in a hole at least 3 inches deep and at least 200 feet away from trails and water sources; a trowel is a basic piece of backpacking equipment. More often, however, the practice of burying human waste is banned or discouraged. Using a portable waste bag (which comes in various forms, available from camping supply vendors) may seem unthinkable at first, but it's really no big deal. Just bring an extra-large zip-top bag for additional insurance against structural failures.

VENTURING AWAY FROM THE CAMPGROUND

If you go for a hike, bike ride, or other excursion into the wilderness, here are some precautions to keep in mind:

- **ALWAYS CARRY FOOD AND WATER,** whether you are planning to go overnight or not. Food will give you energy, help keep you warm, and sustain you in an emergency until help arrives. Bring potable water or treat water by boiling or filtering before drinking from a lake or stream.

- **LET SOMEONE ELSE KNOW WHERE YOU'RE GOING** and when you expect to return. If there's a trailhead register, be sure to sign in.

- **BRING A TRAIL MAP** (kept waterproof in a zip-top bag). In the backcountry, bring a topo map and a compass or a handheld GPS unit with backup batteries.

- **STAY ON DESIGNATED TRAILS.** Hikers most often get lost when venturing off-trail. If the trail has multiple forks, turn back at each and look at it from the other direction, in case you have to retrace your steps. Even on the most clearly marked trails, you may have to stop and consider which direction to head in. If you become disoriented, don't panic. As soon as you think you may be off track, stop, assess your current direction, and then retrace your steps back to the point where you went awry. If you have no idea how to continue, return to the trailhead the way you came in. Should you become completely lost and have no idea of how to return to the trailhead, remaining in place along the trail and waiting for help is most often the best option for adults and always the best option for children.

- **BE CAREFUL WHEN CROSSING STREAMS.** Whether you are fording or crossing on a log, make every step count. If you have any doubt about maintaining your balance on a log, ford the stream instead. When fording, use a trekking pole or stout stick for balance and face upstream as you cross. If a stream seems too deep to ford, turn back. Whatever is on the other side is not worth risking your life.

- **BE CAREFUL AT OVERLOOKS.** The views may be spectacular, but they are also potentially hazardous. Stay away from the edge of outcrops and be absolutely sure of your footing: a misstep can mean a nasty and possibly fatal fall.

- **KNOW THE SYMPTOMS OF HYPOTHERMIA.** Shivering and forgetfulness are the two most common indicators of this insidious killer. Hypothermia can occur at any elevation, even in the summer. Cotton clothing puts you especially at risk, because cotton, when wet, wicks heat away from the body. To prevent hypothermia, dress in layers using synthetic clothing for insulation, use a cap and gloves to reduce heat loss, and protect yourself with waterproof, breathable outerwear. If symptoms arise, take the victim to a shelter, start a fire if you can, give them hot liquids, and put them in dry clothes or a dry sleeping bag.

- **TAKE ALONG YOUR BRAIN.** A cool, calculating mind is the single most important piece of equipment you'll ever need on the trail. Think before you act. Watch your step. Plan ahead. Avoiding accidents before they happen is the best recipe for a rewarding and relaxing hike.

NORTHERN ILLINOIS

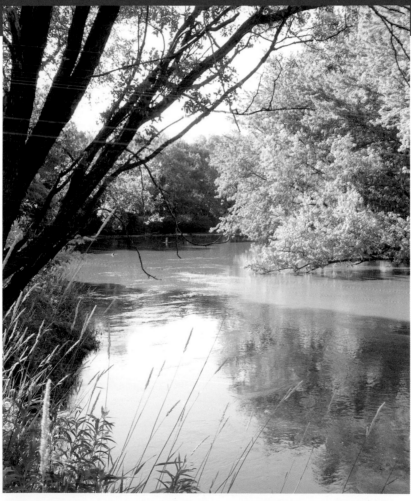

Looking out over the oxbow lake along the Green Trail at Pecatonica River Forest Preserve (see page 32)

Apple River Canyon State Park

Beauty ★★★★★ Privacy ★★★★ Spaciousness ★★★ Quiet ★★★★ Security ★★★★ Cleanliness ★★★★★

Explore this rugged and picturesque canyon carved by the clear waters of the Apple River.

To those of us from the flat farmlands of central Illinois, the topography of Apple River Canyon State Park is a pleasant surprise—can these bluffs and ravines really be part of the Prairie State? Amazingly, yes—this northwest corner of Illinois is something of a geologic island, having escaped the scouring of Ice Age glaciers that leveled hills and filled valleys elsewhere in the state. The same glaciers also blocked the Apple River's outlet, forcing it to carve a new channel southwest. The result is a rugged and picturesque canyon, with towering dolomite cliffs overlooking the clear, bubbling waters of the river below.

The campground, too, is a nice surprise, offering more peace and privacy than I usually expect from drive-in sites at a state park. There are few amenities—no concession or showers, and only a single electric site—but that keeps away the big RVs, and the regulars who camp here year after year are fine with that.

As you enter Apple River Canyon from the east on Canyon Road, pass Walnut Grove youth campground and the park office on the left. At the T-intersection, turn right and head uphill to the entrance to Canyon Ridge Campground on the left.

The layout of Canyon Ridge is similar to that of many state park campgrounds—two loops, with sites situated around the outside and inside of each. What sets this campground apart are the trees: of the 49 sites, many are beautifully secluded from one another by the surrounding woods. Some are accessed by a short grass drive that angles back so you can't even see the site from the road. Even on an average nonholiday weekend, when the campground may be 50%–75% full, you almost feel like you're camping at your own private glade

The beautiful bubbling waters of Apple River

photo by Brian Kapp/Shutterstock

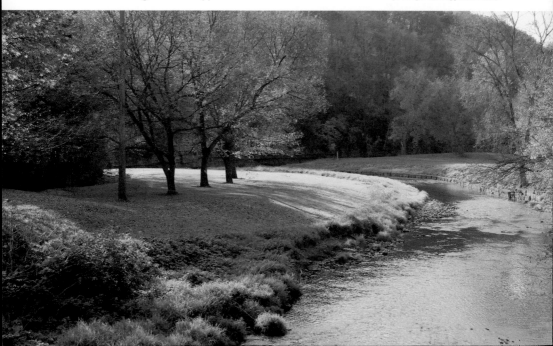

KEY INFORMATION

LOCATION: 8763 East Canyon Road, Apple River, IL 61001

CONTACT: 815-745-3302, bit.ly/AppleRiverIL

OPERATED BY: IDNR

OPEN: Year-round (Canyon Ridge Campground: April 15–October 31, Walnut Grove Campground: year-round)

SITES: Class C: 49

EACH SITE HAS: Picnic table, fire ring, and grate

WHEELCHAIR ACCESS: Restrooms and at least one accessible tent site

ASSIGNMENT: First come, first served; reservations available online

REGISTRATION: Register at the office or with the campground host

AMENITIES: Water spigots, vault toilets

PARKING: At site

FEE: $8/night; $5 reservation fee

ELEVATION: 847'

RESTRICTIONS:

PETS: On leash only

QUIET HOURS: 10 p.m.–7 a.m.

FIRES: In fire rings only

ALCOHOL: Not permitted

VEHICLES: 2 per site

OTHER: 14-day limit; 1 RV and 1 tent, or 2 tents per site; 4 adults or 1 family per site; no swimming or boating

---

in the woods. You will usually find a mix of pop-up campers and tents here, but anything much larger simply wouldn't fit.

In the first loop, containing sites 1–23, I really like sites 2, 3, 8, 10, 11, and 15 for space, shade, and seclusion. Sites 1, 13, and 20 are also good choices, though with less shade. A few others, like 5, 6, and 16–19, are more open and close to the road, so not as private. Note that site 21 in this loop, which has an electric hookup, is used by the campground host, and not available to the public.

The second loop contains sites 24–50; those on the outside of the loop tend to be larger, better shaded, and farther from the road. Here the prize sites are 30 and 50. If you need two adjoining sites, 34 and 36 are a nice combination, with a short trail linking them. You can also reserve any of sites 24–50 online, which I recommend for weekends. Whatever site you pick, head back to the office or campground host (if available) to register.

From November 1–April 15, Canyon Ridge Campground is closed, so winter campers have to use Walnut Grove Campground. Note that Walnut Grove can also be reserved by organized youth groups, so it is wise to call before coming to confirm availability. These 15 or so sites aren't nearly as private as those in the main campground, but during the off-season you'll have few, if any, neighbors here. The campground consists of a single half-circle drive, with parking in the middle. I'd pick a site at the back, away from the road, either to the right as you enter (west) or, even farther back, off the lane to the left (east). Note that the water is shut off during the winter, but there are vault toilets in the middle of the campground.

Hikers can explore the canyon via five excellent trails; some are rugged but well worth the effort to ascend to impressive overlooks. Others take you alongside the clear waters of the Apple River. All of them are 1 mile or less in length and start near the main parking and picnic area south of the campground, just across the river. Pine Ridge, Tower Rock, and River Route Trails are more challenging, while Sunset and Primrose Trails are easier hikes.

Apple River Canyon State Park: Canyon Ridge Campground

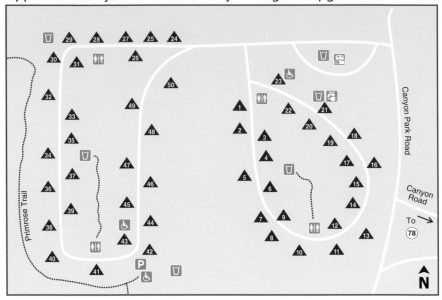

Apple River Canyon State Park: Walnut Grove Campground

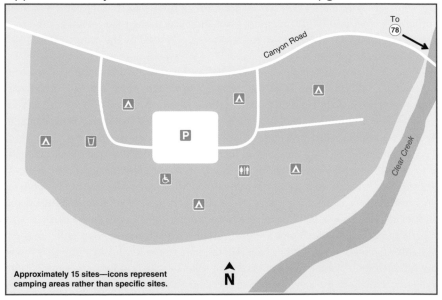

Approximately 15 sites—icons represent camping areas rather than specific sites.

If you want more extensive hiking, head 35 miles or so southwest to the Mississippi River and Mississippi Palisades State Park. This very popular park features 15 miles of hiking trails. The trails in the southern part of the park are steep and rugged in places, leading to some spectacular views of the Mississippi River from the limestone bluffs. Camping is also available, but the large campground is usually full of RVs—I'd rather stay elsewhere, and make this a day trip. This is also one of the few state parks in Illinois where rock climbing and rappelling are permitted—check with the park office for details. To get there from Apple River Canyon, go south from the campground 6.5 miles to US 20. Turn right (west) and go 20 miles to IL 84. Make a left (south) and go 15.3 miles to the north park entrance, on the left. Even if you don't want to hike, the drive along the Mississippi and to the overlooks in the park is well worth it.

GETTING THERE

From Rockford, take US 20 west about 45 miles to IL 78. Turn right (north) and go 6 miles to Canyon Road. Turn left and drive 3.5 miles to the park entrance.

GPS COORDINATES: N42° 26.932'   W90° 03.033'

2

Johnson-Sauk Trail State Recreation Area

Beauty ★★★★ Privacy ★★★ Spaciousness ★★★ Quiet ★★★★ Security ★★★★ Cleanliness ★★★★★

Camp under the tall pines, and enjoy some of the extra conveniences that Johnson-Sauk Trail offers.

More than 300 years ago, the Sauk, among other American Indian tribes, traveled through north-central Illinois on their way from Lake Michigan to the confluence of the Rock and Mississippi Rivers. Today's travelers coming to the Johnson-Sauk Trail State Recreation Area can enjoy the same rolling terrain, along with a scenic lake and some nice conveniences to make their stay a bit more comfortable.

As you enter the park from IL 78, pass the distinctive round barn and take the next right into the Chief Keokuk Campground. You'll immediately be struck by the stately tall pines standing along the road and overshadowing these well-spaced campsites. Stop first at the small parking lot to the left, one of two that serve the 25 nonelectric tent sites. Though these are technically walk-in sites, this campground boasts a gravel access lane between the parking lots. You can drive close to your site only to unload or load, and then park at either end. You get the best of both worlds—you don't have to carry your gear far, and vehicle noise is limited near the campsites.

All these sites are well shaded by the pines, and my favorites are toward the east end. Sites 97 and 98 are popular, offering plenty of space and a great view of the lake—you may

The iconic Ryan's Round Barn is open for tours on select weekends.　　*photo by Karas Hall*

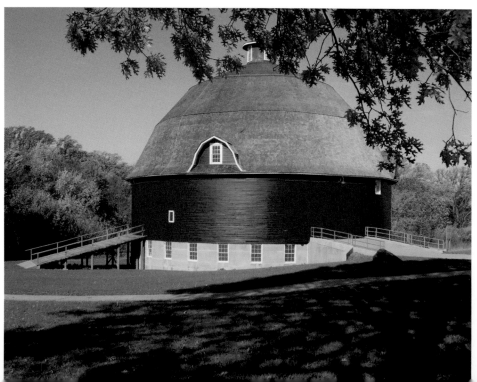

KEY INFORMATION

LOCATION: 28616 Sauk Trail Road, Kewanee, IL 61443

CONTACT: 309-853-2425, bit.ly/JohnsonSaukIL

OPERATED BY: IDNR

OPEN: Year-round

SITES: Class A: 70 electric sites; Class C: 25 walk-in tent sites

EACH SITE HAS: Electricity only in Class A; picnic table, ground grill

WHEELCHAIR ACCESS: Restrooms and at least one accessible tent site.

ASSIGNMENT: First come, first served; reservations available online May–October

REGISTRATION: Set up first, then register with the campground host if available, or park staff will come by

AMENITIES: Water spigots, vault toilets; shower house (no water November–April)

PARKING: At site (Class A); in lot (Class C)

FEE: Class A: $20/night, $30/night holidays; Class C: $8/night; all $2 less when showers are closed

ELEVATION: 781'

RESTRICTIONS:

PETS: On leash only

QUIET HOURS: 10 p.m.–7 a.m.

FIRES: In fire rings only

ALCOHOL: Permitted

VEHICLES: 2 per site

OTHER: 14-day limit; 1 RV and 1 tent, or 2 tents per site; 4 adults or 1 family per site

---

need to arrive early on a weekend to get one of these. Just to the west, 94, 95, and 96 are also nice. Among the others, 78, 82, 83, 84, 87, 88, and 89 are all good choices, sufficiently spacious and set back from the gravel road. The remaining sites are less desirable, being too small, too close to the road, or too crowded with trees.

The 70 electric sites are situated south of the tent area. There's plenty of space between these, but the ones in the largest loop, sites 32–72, aren't as well shaded. If you want electricity, the better sites for tents are along the road past the host. Site 5, 6, 8, or 9 would be my choice, each with plenty of space for setting up a couple of tents.

If some people in your party want a little more roof over their heads, Johnson-Sauk also has the primitive Chief Tecumseh cabin for rent. In May–October it must be reserved online; call for reservations in the off-season.

Whatever you choose, select your site, set up, and then register with the campground host at site 1 or 2, or with park staff, who will come around in the evening if no host is available. All campers can use the very clean, well-maintained shower house, which also includes separate, wheelchair-accessible men's and women's restrooms and showers—a bit of additional privacy not usually found at campgrounds. Note that all water in the campground is turned off from November–April.

The Red Earth Cafe and store, east of the campground, will quickly spoil you. Large and attractive, the restaurant has a full menu and offers everything from bison burgers to vegetarian meals, along with their very popular homemade pie. You can eat inside and enjoy the air-conditioning or dine outside at one of the canopied tables overlooking the lake—watch for the families of ground squirrels. You'll often find a crowd here on weekends, both campers and locals. The store carries food as well as camping and fishing supplies, and you can rent kayaks, johnboats, and paddleboats. The concession's season is April 1–October 1, open daily except for Monday. Call them at 309-853-2784 for details.

If you come on a weekend between May and October, visit Ryan's Round Barn. Constructed between 1908 and 1910 for a Dr. Ryan as part of his cattle farm, this unique building features some labor-saving systems that were innovative for their time. It has been carefully restored by local volunteers, who open the barn for tours on the first, third, and fifth Saturdays of May through October from 1 to 4 p.m. and are available to answer questions.

Johnson-Sauk Trail isn't a hiker's paradise, but if you want to work off the dinner you had at the Red Earth Cafe, it does offer eight short (0.25-mile to 1-mile) well-maintained trails in the day-use area of the park. Cyclists who want more exercise can check out the historic Hennepin Canal State Trail, which runs almost 105 miles along the restored canal towpath. You can connect with the trail at a number of places, but the closest is 6 miles north of Johnson-Sauk off of IL 78, 0.3 mile past I-80. The canal is also an easy canoe route, but you do have to portage around the remaining nonfunctioning locks. For more information and a detailed map, visit the excellent visitor center, open Monday–Friday, 8 a.m.–4 p.m. Call 815-454-2328. To get there, go 12 miles east on I-80 to Exit 45, then head south 1 mile to the sign on the right.

Johnson-Sauk Trail State Recreation Area: Chief Keokuk Campground

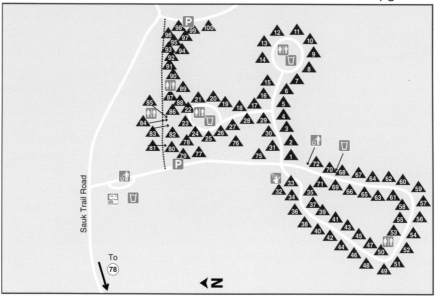

GETTING THERE

From I-80, take Exit 33 onto IL 78 south toward Annawan. Drive 6 miles south, then turn left at the park entrance sign.

From Kewanee, go north on IL 78 (Main Street) 11.5 miles and turn right at the park entrance sign.

GPS COORDINATES: N41° 19.279'   W89° 54.279'

3

Lake Le-Aqua-Na State Park

Beauty ★★★★ Privacy ★★★ Spaciousness ★★★ Quiet ★★★★ Security ★★★★ Cleanliness ★★★★★

Lake Le-Aqua-Na is busy on weekends but is a comfortable place to camp, relax, fish, and swim.

Despite its sound, the name "Lake Le-Aqua-Na" does not come from some American Indian language. It's actually the winning entry from a contest to name the lake, sponsored by the local sportsman's club in 1956: aqua, Latin for "water," stuck in the middle of the name of the nearby town of Lena.

While the name may be a bit unusual, it does reflect the pride that the staff and the local community take in this beautiful park. The 40-acre lake is the centerpiece, and everything around it is well maintained and clean, from the restrooms to the trails and even the campsite fire rings. It's busy on weekends but well worth a visit if you're looking for a comfortable place to camp, relax, and perhaps fish or swim.

Lake Le-Aqua-Na has two campgrounds, and both offer good choices for tent campers. As you enter the park, go straight; soon after the concession you'll come to the first campground, Pine Ridge, on the right. Its 25 sites are used almost exclusively by tent campers— you'll rarely find even a pop-up camper. Each site has a table and a big concrete fire ring.

Most sites are spacious, with more shade and privacy along the outside of the loop, sites 1–13. I like sites 5, 7, and 8 because they're a bit farther back from the road. Site 3 is also good— and near the toilets and water, if that's important. Sites 1 and 2 are a bit close to one another, but if you need two adjoining sites the combination is great because there is plenty of space and trees around. If you don't mind driving to use the showers in Hickory Hill Campground, Pine Ridge is smaller, usually less busy, and just a short walk from the lake and concession.

The only downside of Pine Ridge is that sites 20–24 are the youth group area and are occupied almost every weekend. Before you panic and imagine camping next to a Boy Scout jamboree, however, note that the area is small, and so are most groups that use it. They usually reserve well in advance, so you can call ahead to see if a youth group is expected and how large it might be.

Cross the road from Pine Ridge and walk down the hill to the lake. Follow the trail left along the shore, and you'll come to a secluded bench where you can fish or just sit and enjoy the view—the sunrise is nice from here. Continue around the bend to reach the concession building. At the time of writing, the park did not have a concessionaire to run the snack bar and boat rental service here. Check with the park for updated information.

Lake Le-Aqua-Na
photo by Terri Waller Wachtveitl

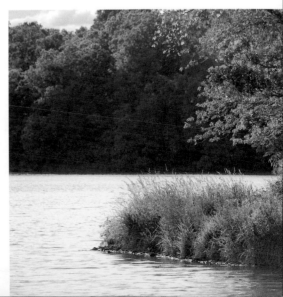

KEY INFORMATION

LOCATION: 8542 North Lake Road, Lena, IL 61048

CONTACT: 815-369-4282, bit.ly/LeAquaNaIL

OPERATED BY: IDNR

OPEN: Year-round

SITES: At Pine Ridge, 1 Class A and 24 Class B; at Hickory Hill, 142 Class A and 11 Class B

EACH SITE HAS: Electricity at Class A only; picnic table and fire ring

WHEELCHAIR ACCESS: Restrooms and at least one accessible tent site

ASSIGNMENT: First come, first served; most sites are reservable May 1–October 31

REGISTRATION: Set up and park staff will come by

AMENITIES: Water spigots, vault toilets; shower house (no water November–April)

PARKING: At site

FEE: Class A: $20/night, $30/night holidays; Class B: $10/night; all sites $2 less when showers are closed; $5 reservation fee

ELEVATION: 926'

RESTRICTIONS:

PETS: On leash only

QUIET HOURS: 10 p.m.–7 a.m.

FIRES: In fire rings only

ALCOHOL: Not permitted

VEHICLES: 2 per site

OTHER: 14-day limit; 1 RV and 1 tent, or 2 tents per site; 4 adults or 1 family per site

---

Farther down the road from Pine Ridge is Hickory Hill Campground. All but 11 of these 153 sites have electrical hookups, so this is RV territory. However, if you are lucky enough to snag one, the four nonelectric tent sites on the left as you drive in are great. Each is situated well back in the surrounding woods, but you can drive on the grass right to your site. Sites 151 and 152 are particularly private, nestled in a grove of trees but within a short walk of the shower building.

The other seven nonelectric sites are 1–7, located on a hilltop to the right as you enter the campground. These are fairly spacious but wide open with little shade. If you want electricity, you'll probably find a bit more privacy and shade at the back, around sites 86 and 87. You can expect this campground to be busy on an average weekend. The campground hosts have a stack of brochures on both the park and surrounding attractions.

Fishing is popular at Lake Le-Aqua-Na. In addition to containing typical Illinois species like crappie, bluegill, channel catfish, and largemouth bass, the lake is just far enough north to accommodate northern pike. Kids will enjoy the small, free swimming beach near the park entrance, and adults will at least find it a good place to cool off. If you want chlorinated swimming, check out Splash Land water park in Lena, which has a couple of pools, an awesome waterslide, and minigolf. Call 815-369-9165 for more information.

GETTING THERE

From Rockford, take US 20 west about 40 miles to IL 73. Turn right (north) and drive 1.7 miles into Lena. Turn left on Lena Street, and go 0.4 mile to Freedom Street. Turn right and head 3 miles north to the park entrance, on the left.

GPS COORDINATES: N42° 25.240'   W89° 49.451'

Lake Le-Aqua-Na State Park: Pine Ridge Campground

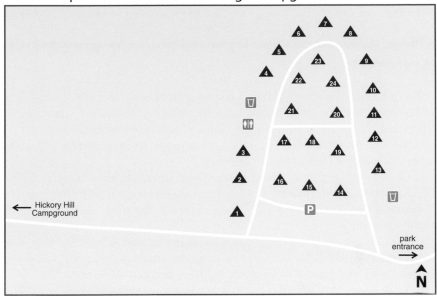

Lake Le-Aqua-Na State Park: Hickory Hill Campground

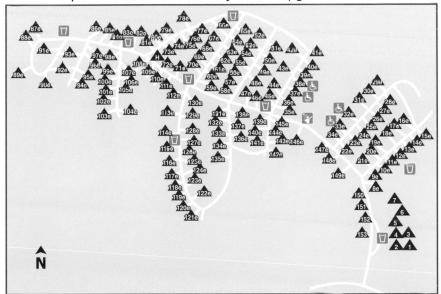

4

Loud Thunder Forest Preserve

Beauty ★★★★★ Privacy ★★★★ Spaciousness ★★★ Quiet ★★★★ Security ★★★★★ Cleanliness ★★★★★

Lake George, nestled amid the surrounding forested hills, is a tranquil spot for boating, hiking, and camping.

At 1,621 acres, Loud Thunder is the largest and most picturesque of the Rock Island County Forest Preserves. There are miles of multiuse trails, beautiful views of the Mississippi River, and 167-acre Lake George, nestled amid the forested hills. With the Quad Cities just to the north, Loud Thunder is popular on weekends, but five separate campgrounds with a total of 116 sites offer plenty of choices for tent campers.

All campers must go first to the office, where you register before setting up. Go down the hill, across the dam, and take the first left. From May–Labor Day, office hours are Friday and Saturday, 8 a.m.–8 p.m. and 8 a.m.–7 p.m. the rest of the week; check the website for hours the rest of the year.

The first campground you'll see as you enter Loud Thunder is Silva, 0.6 mile from IL 92 on the left. Silva offers 19 sites located along a ridge stretching toward Lake George. In recent years staff have planted more brush and trees between them, providing more privacy. Those on the right as you enter (west) overlook a small valley, while those on the east have trees behind them. Sites S8 and S9 at the end are a bit more spacious and set back from the road, as are sites S11–S15 on the east.

Riverview Campground features 11 campsites at river's edge with beautiful vistas.
photo by Kim Walker

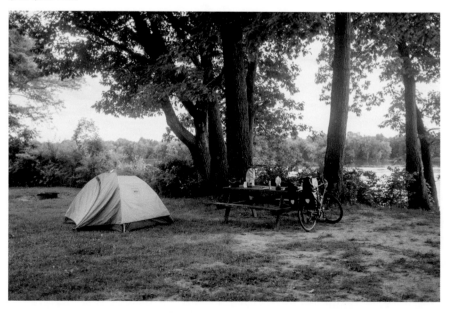

KEY INFORMATION

LOCATION: 19406 Loud Thunder Road, Illinois City, IL 61259

CONTACT: 309-795-1040, bit.ly/LoudThunderIL

OPERATED BY: Rock Island County Forest Preserve District

OPEN: April 1–October 31 (weather permitting)

SITES: White Oak Campground (electric and water hookups): 26 sites; other campgrounds (nonelectric): 90 sites

EACH SITE HAS: Picnic table, fire ring

WHEELCHAIR ACCESS: Restrooms

ASSIGNMENT: First come, first served; reservations available online

REGISTRATION: At park office

AMENITIES: Water spigots, vault and flush toilets, shower house

PARKING: At site

FEE: White Oak Campground: $20/night; other campgrounds: $15/$16/night ($2 less for county residents, $3 less for senior citizens); $3.50 reservation fee

ELEVATION: 722'

RESTRICTIONS:

PETS: On leash only

QUIET HOURS: 10 p.m.–7 a.m.

FIRES: In fire rings only

ALCOHOL: Permitted

VEHICLES: 2 per site

OTHER: 14-day limit; 1 RV or 1 tent per site

The entrance to the Riverview Campground loop is 0.25 mile past Silva on the right, then 0.3 mile down the hill to the Mississippi River. There's not much shade or privacy, but 11 of these 30 sites (R20–R30) offer impressive vistas right at the riverside. You're actually not even looking across the entire width of the Mississippi here, only about 0.25 mile to Andalusia Island in the middle of the river. The sites at the eastern edge (R29 and R30) are a bit farther from traffic, but this campground is the most popular nonelectric one at Loud Thunder, so don't count on solitude most weekends. All campers can use the brand-new shower house here, or the one at White Oak Campground.

Head down the hill from the Riverview entrance, across the dam, and turn left at the park office. The left fork leads to the boat ramp, the right to White Oak, Indian Meadows, and Horse Corral Campgrounds. White Oak has 26 electric sites for RVs only, no tents allowed. Adjacent Indian Meadows has 20 sites ranged along a ridge with brush and trees between them. Sites on the east (right as you enter) are a bit more spacious and overlook the lake below. Note that sites I1–I3 and I7 are designated for two camping units—you pay for and can set up two tents. I like site I14, on the loop at the end of the road, with its surrounding trees.

At the end of the road, Horse Corral is the least used of the campgrounds, and fortunately 12 of its 21 sites are open to all campers, not just equestrians. Most sites here are close to the road and in an open field with little shade. To reach the most secluded site in all of Loud Thunder (my favorite), turn right onto the gravel road as you enter the campground and continue about 600 feet along the edge of the field. You'll come to two-unit site H1, situated all by itself in a wooded opening. If you didn't have a campground map (or this book), you wouldn't even know it existed. Except for the designated two-unit sites, all sites at Loud Thunder are limited to one camping unit, either a tent or an RV. You can reserve any site online at sunrisereservations.com for an additional $3.50.

Loud Thunder offers hikers, mountain bikers, and equestrians diverse opportunities to explore the forested ridges surrounding Lake George and the bottomlands along the Mississippi. The trails north of Loud Thunder Road are limited to foot traffic, while most of the trails to the south are designated multiuse. For an easier hike with wonderful views of the river, head east from Riverview Campground on the east branch of Hauberg Trail. You can hike the entire 1.2 miles to the parking lot on I-92, then return via part of the Sac-Fox Trail. More challenging is the southern portion of Sac-Fox, about 8 miles total, including a 4.6-mile loop that begins at Horse Corral Campground. This section is popular with mountain bikers as well. For detailed trail maps, check the excellent and informative Forest Preserve District website: ricfpd.org.

Fishing and boating are popular at Loud Thunder, both on Lake George and the Mississippi. Since boats on the lake are limited to those with trolling motors, it's quiet too. The park office rents one- and two-person kayaks, four- and eight-person pontoon boats, and johnboats, and it sells bait, tackle, and snacks.

Loud Thunder is named after the son of Sauk Indian leader Black Hawk, whose people occupied the area from about 1750–1831, when they were forced across the Mississippi by encroaching settlement. His courageous but ill-fated war in 1832 to reclaim his home village eventually made him a local hero. Black Hawk State Historic Site on Rock Island provides a fascinating overview of his life and the culture of the Sauk and Fox tribes. Check blackhawkpark.org for more information.

Loud Thunder Forest Preserve: Silva Campground

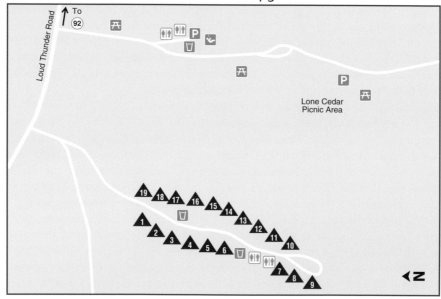

Loud Thunder Forest Preserve: Riverview Campground

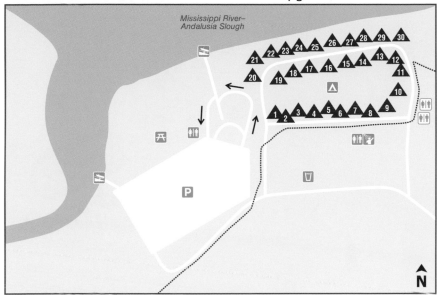

Loud Thunder Forest Preserve:
White Oak and Indian Meadows Campgrounds

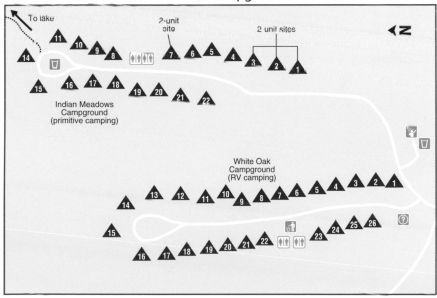

Loud Thunder Forest Preserve: Horse Corral Campground

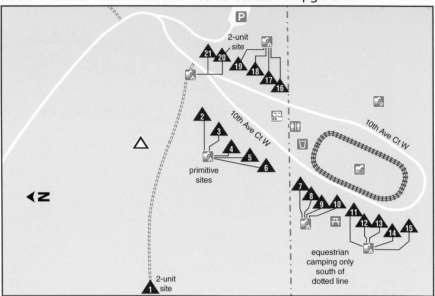

GETTING THERE

From I-280, take Exit 11 onto IL 92 W toward Andalusia. Drive 1.5 miles south and turn right, following IL 92. Go 12 miles west through Andalusia to Loud Thunder Road and turn right into the forest preserve.

GPS COORDINATES: N41° 25.911'   W90° 49.247'

5

Marengo Ridge Conservation Area

Beauty ★★★★ Privacy ★★★★★ Spaciousness ★★★ Quiet ★★★★ Security ★★★★★ Cleanliness ★★★★★

What a surprise—wonderfully isolated tent camping within striking distance of Chicago!

When I plan an Illinois camping getaway, my mind usually gravitates south—or east, west, or northwest—in fact, to any corner of the state but the northeast, aka Chicago. I'm not enamored of expressways and malls, and "big city" and "camping" just don't go together for me. However, not many miles from the busy northwest suburbs, you'll find Marengo Ridge, a superb McHenry County conservation area that doesn't look a bit like Chicago and offers wonderfully isolated tent camping.

As you enter the conservation area off IL 23, head straight back to the Thomas Woods Campground entrance and stop first at the trailer to register. Here you'll also find trail maps and can purchase firewood and ice. This southern loop of the campground has 18 sites that accommodate RVs, though only two, sites 0 and 4, have electric hookups. Tent campers can also use these sites.

Drive past sites 1–3 and turn left to enter the tent-only area with its 29 beautifully wooded sites. All of these sites have a table, a fire ring with a grill, and a flat, raised tent pad bordered by landscaping timbers and filled with fine-crushed gravel. (You're not required to pitch your tent on the pad, however.) Most are well shaded under a mix of pine and hardwoods. You can pull into 7 of the sites, but far better for privacy are any of the 22 walk-in sites, which have been carefully laid out in separate sections of just a few sites each. The result is that even on busy weekends the campground doesn't feel crowded, and at many sites you'll find yourself nicely secluded from neighbors by the surrounding trees and brush.

View south from the overlook atop Marengo Ridge *courtesy of McHenry County Conservation District*

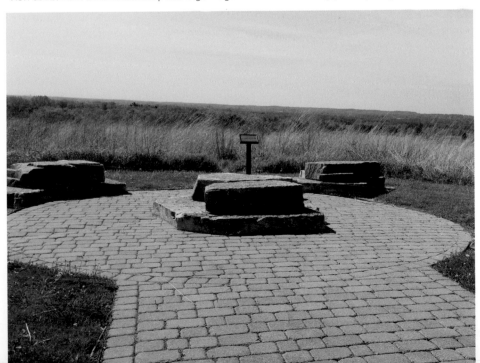

KEY INFORMATION

LOCATION: 2411 N. IL 23, Marengo, IL 60152

CONTACT: 815-338-6223, bit.ly/MarengoRidgeIL

OPERATED BY: McHenry County Conservation District

OPEN: May 1–October 31, Friday and Saturday nights only, plus holidays

SITES: 29 tent sites (22 walk-in); 18 RV sites (2 electric)

EACH SITE HAS: Picnic table, fire ring

WHEELCHAIR ACCESS: Restrooms and at least one accessible tent site

ASSIGNMENT: First come, first served; reservations available online

REGISTRATION: Register at the check-in trailer

AMENITIES: Water spigots, vault toilets

PARKING: At site; at lot for walk-in sites

FEE: $12/night nonelectric ($18 out-of-county residents); $22/night electric ($33 out-of-county residents); $2/night holiday surcharge ($5 out-of-county residents); $2 reservation fee

ELEVATION: 893'

RESTRICTIONS:

PETS: On leash only

QUIET HOURS: 10 p.m.–7 a.m.

FIRES: In fire rings only

ALCOHOL: Not within 100 feet of a parking area

VEHICLES: 1 per site (tent area)

OTHER: Check-in by 7 p.m.; no amplified music; 3-day maximum stay (2-day extension possible); 8 people per site except for larger families

You'll first pass sites 18–27 along the lower road. These are older and not quite as spread out as those on the ridge above, but there are still some excellent options here. In the first set of walk-ins, site 18 is the farthest from the others, though it is also right along a hiking trail. Site 21 is also in a pretty spot by itself.

Turn right past site 27 and head uphill to the newer tent sites. Most of the walk-in sites here are well separated from one another, with just enough distance between you and the parking lot so you're not disturbed by vehicle lights and noises. The best are those farthest from their respective parking areas: sites 29, 30, 34, 36, 44, and 46. If you and a friend need a pair of sites, 36 and 37 are adjoining, linked by a short trail. My favorite is 44, all by itself down a short trail, about 150 feet from parking, and well worth the walk. If you prefer a pull-in site, 39, 40, and 42 are good choices.

With its proximity to Chicago, Marengo Ridge is popular, and it's unfortunately only open for camping on Friday and Saturday nights (as well as Memorial Day, July Fourth, and Labor Day holidays). It's wise to make reservations online no later than the Wednesday before at noon.

The terrain around Marengo Ridge can best be described as undulating, the result of successive waves of glaciers that deposited mounds of sand and gravel as they melted and receded. The forest preserve itself rests atop part of the Marengo Moraine, a ridge that marks the westernmost limits of the Wisconsin ice sheet and stretches from the state line south about 40 miles. The resulting panorama can best be appreciated from the observation area south of the preserve entrance, where you can look out for miles over the rolling prairie. Look for the interpretive sign that describes what you're seeing and puts it all in geologic perspective.

You can further explore Marengo Ridge through the 5-mile network of hiking trails. The southern loop descends into the valley from the observation point, and the northern loops wind through a mix of pine, oak, and hickory forest, up and down the hills, and past intermittent streams.

If Marengo Ridge is the best place to tent camp in McHenry County, then Moraine Hills State Park is a prime choice for hiking and biking. This 2,200-acre park east of Marengo is also characterized by glacially formed topography—rolling hills, marshes, bogs, and 48-acre Lake Defiance, one of the few glacial lakes in Illinois that has remained largely undeveloped. Over 10 miles of well-maintained trails traverse the park in four connected loops, all paved or surfaced with crushed limestone, and very popular with cyclists. Whether you are on bike or on foot, keep an eye out for the incredible diversity of plant and animal life present, including one of Illinois's largest colonies of rare carnivorous pitcher plants.

You can also fish along the Fox River or from the boardwalk at Lake Defiance, and boat rental and snacks are available at the Fish Tales Concession from April–mid-October. To get there from Marengo Ridge, go 2 miles south on IL 23 to IL 176 (Telegraph Street) in Marengo. Turn left, proceed 22 miles east, over the Fox River, and turn left onto River Road. The park entrance is 2 miles north. Call 815-385-1624 or check bit.ly/MoraineHillsIL for more information.

Marengo Ridge Conservation Area: Thomas Woods Campground

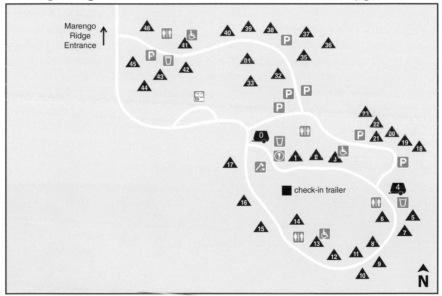

GETTING THERE

From I-90 (Northwest Tollway), take Exit 36 and go 9 miles north on US 20 to Marengo. Turn right onto IL 23 (State Street). Go 2.5 miles north to forest preserve entrance on the right.

GPS COORDINATES: N42° 17.037'   W88° 36.420'

6

Pecatonica River Forest Preserve

Beauty ★★★★★ Privacy ★★★ Spaciousness ★★★★ Quiet ★★★★ Security ★★★★★ Cleanliness ★★★★★

This quiet forest campground sees the least traffic of any in Winnebago County.

As I've searched Illinois for interesting, quiet, less well-known places to camp, I've come to appreciate the hidden gems managed by many of the 102 counties that make up the Prairie State. State parks are easy to find online, and the national forest campgrounds in southern Illinois are well known. But the campgrounds found in county conservation areas and forest preserves are often unknown outside their local area, and many see few campers.

The Pecatonica River Forest Preserve is just such a place. It's the smallest of the four campgrounds in the excellent Winnebago County system, and the only one without electric hookups. Consequently, it also has the least campground traffic, and some weekends you may have the place all to yourself.

As you enter the forest preserve off Judd Road, turn right toward the campground. Stop first at the information board at the entrance, where you self-register. You can also purchase firewood here on an honor system, at $7 per bundle.

The campground consists of a single loop, with 15 primitive sites arranged around it, each with a picnic table and a fire ring. There's a single set of vault toilets, and water spigots in several places. The sites at the back of the loop (5–8) and on the west (10–15) have the most shade and space. My favorites are 14 and 15, where you can camp beneath mature oaks with plenty of room to spread out. All sites are first come, first served, so pick your favorite and settle in. When I camped there on a beautiful June weekend, only one other site was occupied, and it was a peaceful, quiet evening, with birdsong and a firefly light show for entertainment.

This observation platform overlooks the oxbow lake along the Green Trail.

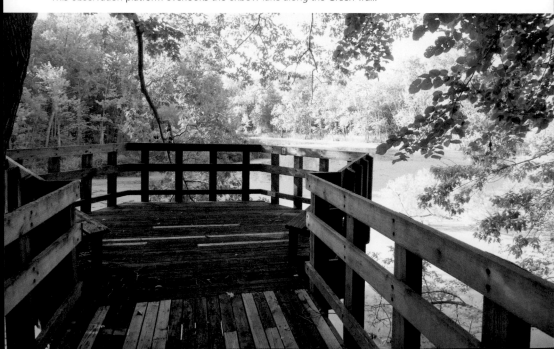

The forest preserve is bounded on the east by the slow-moving, meandering Pecatonica River. (The name comes from two Algonquin words probably meaning "slow water.") In the course of its wanderings, the Pecatonica has left several oxbow lakes and wetlands scattered among the woods, creating an ideal habitat for all sorts of wildlife. Take time to explore via some of the 9.8 miles of hiking trails laid out in three color-coded sections. The Green Trail is the shortest, and starts near the large pavilion at the preserve entrance. Check out the interesting 130-year-old stone barn along the way, then cross the road south. The trail continues to an observation deck overlooking a large oxbow lake. Bring binoculars, and stop here to look and listen carefully—you may hear or see a variety of birds and amphibians, including leopard frogs, spring peepers, and even sandhill cranes who stop over during their spring and fall migrations. The trail descends to follow the river for a distance, then returns to Judd Road. You'll find excellent trail maps to download on the preserve's website.

The trailhead for the Blue Trail is located just 0.5 mile south on Judd Road (which becomes Brick School Road when it curves to the right). Take the first left past the curve, and look for the parking area on the left. The 2-mile trail winds through prairie and grassland, and leads to an abandoned limestone quarry where careful eyes can spot fossils. (If you want to avoid the hike, drive past the trailhead parking directly to the quarry.)

Winnebago County features quite a few other interesting outdoor places to explore, even without venturing into the big city of Rockford itself. Pecatonica Wetlands Forest Preserve is 5 miles southwest, with 10 miles of hiking trails. Seward Bluffs Forest Preserve is another 5 miles south, and one of the most scenic places to hike in the area. About 8 miles of trails explore the woodlands, prairie, and bluffs surrounding Grove Creek. Severson Dells Forest Preserve is 19 miles southwest, and especially worth visiting for kids. They'll enjoy exploring the Grove, a natural play area, and Severson hosts a wide range of special environmental education events for kids and families, including nature programs, guided hikes, and even guided canoe ventures on portions of the Kishwaukee River. Trail maps, event schedules, and other information about all these places can be found on the Winnebago County Forest Preserve District website: winnebagoforest.org.

The Pecatonica is a muddy river, but nonetheless popular with local canoeists. There is unfortunately at present no outfitter renting canoes or leading trips on it. Kishwaukee Canoe in Rockford provides canoe/kayak rental and shuttle service for the clear, broad, smooth-flowing Kishwaukee River. Call 815-968-0711 or check kishwaukeecanoe.com for more information.

Pecatonica River Forest Preserve Campground

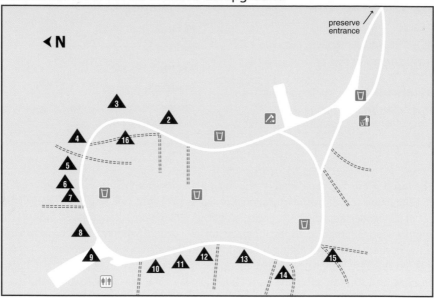

GETTING THERE

From I-39 at Rockford, take US 20 W 13.9 miles to Winnebago Road. Turn right, proceed 5.7 miles to IL 70 (Trask Bridge Road), and turn left. Go 4.3 miles to Judd Road and turn left. The preserve entrance will be 1.3 miles ahead on the right.

GPS COORDINATES: N42° 21.518′   W89° 19.277′

7

Sugar River Forest Preserve

Beauty ★★★★ Privacy ★★★ Spaciousness ★★★★★ Quiet ★★★★ Security ★★★★ Cleanliness ★★★★

Camp, hike, or canoe along the serene and isolated banks of the lazy Sugar River.

One of the most serene and isolated rivers in northern Illinois is the Sugar, which meanders lazily from Wisconsin south toward Rockford. Its waters are clear, flowing over sandy soil, along low banks, and by sandy bluffs. The surrounding countryside is mostly unspoiled by development, thanks largely to Winnebago County, which has set aside 529 acres along its banks to form the Sugar River Forest Preserve. Sugar River's campground is popular, but there are also good spots for tent camping along the river.

As you enter on Forest Preserve Road, take the right fork toward the campground. Pine Tree campground has 70 electric sites, situated around a single loop within a large grove of pines, as the name suggests. The sites aren't secluded, but they are spacious compared to those at most park RV campgrounds, in addition to being flat and fairly well shaded. The sites around the outside of the loop (sites 32–70) are deeper and roomier, and there are more trees toward the back—site 46 is the best here. This campground is about half to three-quarters full most nonholiday weekends.

Much more secluded and spacious, but less shaded, are the 12 walk-in sites along the Sugar River. Go left at the campground entrance, and you'll come to the small parking area, with vault toilets and a water spigot. From here it's an easy, flat walk of about 400–800 feet

Bird banding at nearby Colored Sands Forest Preserve   *courtesy of CheepShot/Flickr*

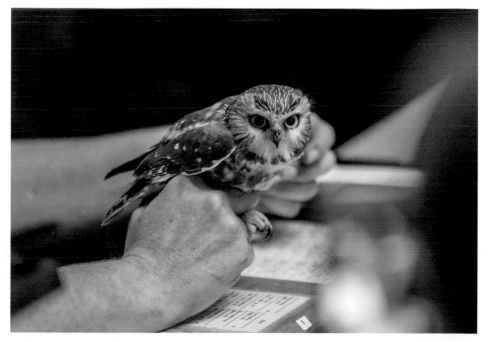

KEY INFORMATION

LOCATION: 10127 Forest Preserve Road, Durand, IL 61024

CONTACT: 815-877-6100, bit.ly/SugarRiverIL

OPERATED BY: Winnebago County Forest Preserve District

OPEN: Mid-April–mid-November

SITES: 12 walk-in sites and 70 vehicle-access sites

EACH SITE HAS: Picnic table, fire ring; electric in main campground only

WHEELCHAIR ACCESS: Restrooms and at least one accessible electric site

ASSIGNMENT: First come, first served; reservations available online for 21 vehicle-access sites

REGISTRATION: Set up and park staff will come by (May–October); in absence of camp host, use self-registration station

AMENITIES: Water spigots, vault toilets; shower house in main campground only

PARKING: At campsite or in lot

FEE: Walk-in sites: $23/night; Regular sites: $25/night (both $10 less for Winnebago County residents); $8 electric hookup

ELEVATION: 807'

RESTRICTIONS:

PETS: On leash only

QUIET HOURS: 10 p.m.–8 a.m.

FIRES: In fire rings only

ALCOHOL: Permitted

VEHICLES: 2 per site

OTHER: 14-day limit; 3 tents per site; set up and register by 10 p.m.; no gathering of downed wood

---

to any of the sites, and you can bring a wagon to haul your gear, if you want. This area is also popular—about three-quarters full most weekends.

Walk east from the parking lot to site 10 on the river—sites 4–9 are to the left, 11 and 12 to the right, and 1–3 are away from the river, accessed by a short trail from site 7. These are all situated on sandy, grass-covered soil, with no brush or trees between them. Each has a table and a fire ring, and sites 4–12 are just a few steps from the riverbank. On the left, I like site 4 because it's at the end of the row, so neighbors won't be walking by to get to their sites, and it has some trees around. Site 1 is more secluded and wooded, though not on the river. Site 6 also has some shade.

Farthest from the other sites is the combination of sites 11 and 12, which afford lots of room to spread out. Since the forest preserve allows up to three tents per site, these would be ideal for a small group. Wherever you choose, set up and park staff will come by to register you. Unfortunately, walk-in camping fees do not include use of the shower house in the main campground.

Because of their location, these sites may flood in the early spring. Also, when I was there, the mosquitoes were terrible, even in the middle of the day. However, staff said there'd been a lot of flooding recently, and consequently they were much worse than usual. If you're hoping to come in the spring to midsummer, call first for conditions and bring bug spray.

The best way to see the river is by canoe, and there are numerous access points along its length, from Wisconsin down to where it joins with the muddier but equally scenic Pecatonica. Note that the river is sometimes too high or low to canoe safely and also tricky to navigate because of deadfall. However, there are no outfitters serving the Sugar in Illinois, so if you don't have your own canoe and means of shuttling, you'll have to be content exploring on foot. Sugar River Forest Preserve offers 6 miles of hiking trails, and Colored Sands Forest Preserve, to the north across Yale Road, adds another 2-mile loop. The latter is so named because of the unique 40-foot multicolored sandy bluff on the east bank, near a bend in the river. The hike from the entrance to the bluff is about 0.75 mile. To get there from Sugar River, go east on Yale Road to Hauley Road, turn left, continue 0.5 mile north to Haas Road, turn left again, and go 1 mile to the forest preserve entrance, on the left. Excellent trail maps for all the county forest preserves can be found on the district website: wcfpd.org.

Colored Sands is also home to the Sand Bluff Bird Observatory, which offers visitors a rare opportunity to participate in banding migrating birds. On spring and fall weekends, volunteers use large mesh nets to trap birds, then gently measure their wingspans and attach an aluminum band to the leg, allowing their travels to be monitored. Over the years, they have banded more than 85,000 birds of 150-plus species. Large maps with pins indicate where those birds were later spotted throughout the Americas. Visitors are welcome and can help release birds. Banding takes place March–May and September–November, and the annual Birdfest on Mother's Day weekend includes activities for kids, raptor demonstrations, special exhibits, and food vendors. Call the forest preserve for more information, or check sandbluff.org.

Sugar River Forest Preserve Campgrounds

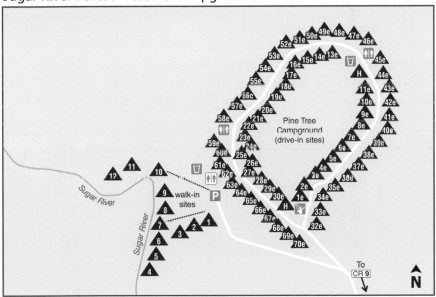

GETTING THERE

From I-39, take Exit 3 and head west on Rockton Road (CR 9) 8 miles to Forest Preserve Road. Turn right and drive 4.5 miles to the Sugar River Forest Preserve entrance.

GPS COORDINATES: N42° 27.802'   W89° 14.144'

8

Woodford State Fish and Wildlife Area

Beauty ★★★ Privacy ★★★ Spaciousness ★★★ Quiet ★★★★★ Security ★★★★ Cleanliness ★★★★

You can watch blue herons catch their dinner, fish for your own dinner, or simply relax at this small primitive campground near the Illinois River.

Woodford State Fish and Wildlife Area covers 2,900 acres, more than 80% of which is water—not surprising, since the Illinois River valley here north of Peoria is broad and low-lying, and the river spreads out to create large, shallow backwater lakes. The balance of the acreage is bottomland forest and seasonal wetlands, creating a combination that's a welcome haven for waterfowl. Equally inviting to tent campers is the small primitive camp-ground near the river, where you can watch blue herons catch their dinner, fish for your own dinner, or just relax.

The camping area consists of a single loop of about 25 unnumbered grassy sites, each with a ground grill and a table. The sites around the outside of the loop on the east are adjacent to a large field that offers plenty of space for spreading out or throwing a football. There isn't a lot of shade, but the first two sites on the east have some pines, and those at the back of the loop are the best-shaded and nicest sites. The west side of the loop is bordered by a man-made fishing channel that connects to the river. You'll find vault toilets

Looking out over the Illinois River   *photo by Karas Hall*

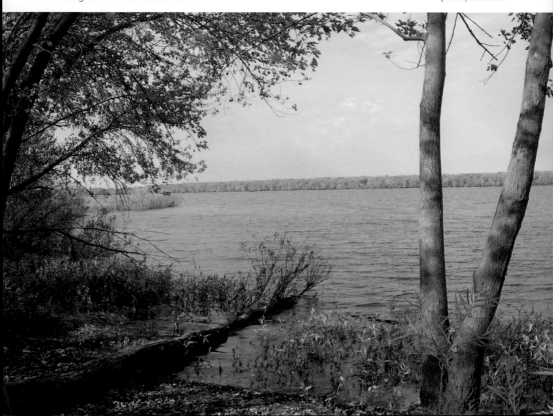

KEY INFORMATION

LOCATION: 524 Conservation Lane, Lowpoint, IL 61545

CONTACT: Marshall SF&WA, 309-246-8351, bit.ly/Woodford-IL

OPERATED BY: IDNR

OPEN: April 1–October 1

SITES: 25 Class C sites

EACH SITE HAS: Picnic table, ground grill

WHEELCHAIR ACCESS: Not designated

ASSIGNMENT: First come, first served

REGISTRATION: Register with the campground host or set up and park staff will come by

AMENITIES: Water spigots, vault toilets

PARKING: At campsite

FEE: $8/night

ELEVATION: 444'

RESTRICTIONS:

PETS: On leash only

QUIET HOURS: 10 p.m.–7 a.m.

FIRES: In fire rings only

ALCOHOL: Permitted

VEHICLES: 2 per site

OTHER: 14-day limit; 4 adults or 1 family per site

and a water spigot at the end of the loop. The only RV you'll probably see is the one in the middle of the loop, belonging to the campground host. Register with the host; if no one is there, park staff will come by.

There's nothing fancy or particularly scenic about the campground itself. What is attractive is the quiet. Outside of waterfowl-hunting season (when the campground is closed), not many people make the 1-mile drive off of IL 26 to this secluded spot along the river. In April and May, a very busy weekend might see half the sites occupied; during the summer and early fall, chances are good it will just be you and the campground host. Note that the campground is only open from April 1–September 30.

You can't see the Illinois River from your campsite, but you can walk or drive about 0.25 mile to it, and the view is impressive. The river spreads out across the lowlands to form shallow Goose Lake, and the opposite shore is about 2 miles away at this point. There's a boat ramp and a fish-cleaning station here. There are also three hiking trails starting at the end of the campground and extending about 1 mile north. The hiking is easy, with trails following along the tops of the levees created to manage seasonal flooding of the wetlands. The westernmost one, Goose Lake Trail, offers the best views of the river. You can hike that out, and pick up Wood Duck Trail for the return trip, making a 2-mile loop.

Bird-watchers like this area along the Illinois River because of the abundance of waterfowl, raptors, and many other species. You'll certainly see wood ducks, Canada geese, blue herons, egrets, swans, red-tailed hawks, owls, and, if you're fortunate, bald eagles. They're more common in the winter, but recently a nesting pair of bald eagles was located not far from Woodford, just off a trail. Check with park staff for their current status.

Marshall State Fish and Wildlife Area is just 5.8 miles north of Woodford on IL 26, also right on the Illinois River. There's a small campground there, and unlike Woodford's, it's open year-round. This spot tends to attract more campers, probably because it has 21 electric sites and is visible from the highway. Some of the electric sites on the west side (notably sites 5–11) are well shaded and offer a beautiful view of the river. There are also eight sandy nonelectric sites bunched together, and toilets and a water spigot are nearby. The biggest drawback to camping at Marshall is the highway noise—the campsites are barely 150 feet from IL 26. A fence separates the electric sites from the highway, but nothing shields the nonelectric ones.

Just across IL 26, to the east, the land quickly rises some 200 feet in impressive wooded bluffs. Marshall includes 3.5 miles of fairly rugged trails that traverse this upland oak-hickory forest, winding along the bluffs and up and down the ravines. I don't think many people take advantage of these beautiful trails. I suggest hiking the loop clockwise—start with the moderate 0.5-mile walk down to the bluffs on Walnut Trail, then take your time enjoying the views along the 0.75-mile Bluff Trail, and finish getting a workout on the 2-mile Ravine Run Trail, with its staircases and bridges. To get to the trailhead, go 1 mile north of the Marshall entrance, then turn right onto Richland Road. Continue 0.5 mile to Blue Heron Road and turn right. Go 0.6 mile to the trailhead parking on the right. Pick up a trail map at the Marshall office, north of the campground, on the east side of the highway.

Woodford State Fish and Wildlife Area Campground

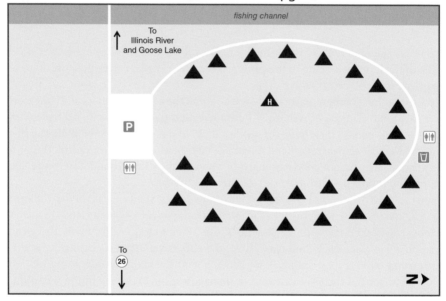

GETTING THERE

From I-74 at East Peoria, take Exit 95 to IL 116 and head north 5 miles to IL 26. Take the left fork onto IL 26, and go 12.6 miles to Conservation Lane. Turn left, and drive 0.9 mile to the campground entrance.

From I-39, take Exit 35 to IL 17, then head west 18.3 miles to IL 26 in Lacon. Turn left, go 10.5 miles south to Conservation Lane, make a right, and drive 0.9 mile to the campground entrance.

GPS COORDINATES: N40° 52.742'   W89° 27.126'

CENTRAL ILLINOIS

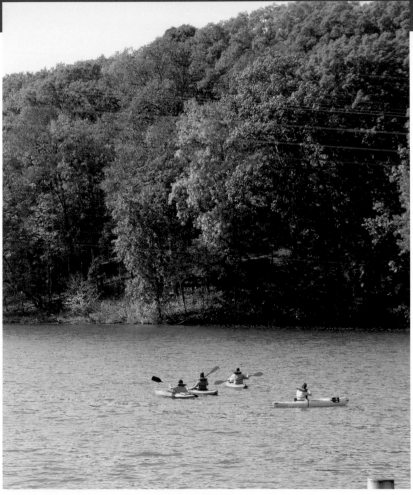

Rent a kayak at the concession and explore the lake at Lincoln Trail (see page 70).

9

⚕ Argyle Lake State Park

Beauty ★★★★★ Privacy ★★★★ Spaciousness ★★★ Quiet ★★★★ Security ★★★★ Cleanliness ★★★★★

Families will love the visitor center and variety of naturalist-led programs.

I really wanted to include Argyle Lake State Park in the first edition of this book. There was so much to like about it: a gorgeous 93-acre lake surrounded by wooded hills, a cool little visitor center with kid-friendly exhibits and activities, and a great restaurant. But the road to the best area for tent campers was closed at that time, waiting on state funding to repair it. Well, the road is fixed, the campgrounds open, the restaurant even better than before, and this 1,700-acre park is well worth a visit.

Argyle Lake is circled by an almost 6-mile loop road, with three different campgrounds situated around it. From the park entrance, take the third right to Twisted Oaks Campground, with its 85 Class A electric sites. Here you'll see the campground host's site near the entrance, where you can register, and the recently renovated shower house, which all campers can use. These sites are great for RVs, but shade and privacy are limited.

Big Oaks Campground, on the opposite side of the lake, has 23 Class B electric sites, and 12 Class C nonelectric sites. This campground is not as busy as Twisted Oaks. Of the Class C sites, C1–C10, at the north end of the campground, don't offer much privacy, but C6 and C7 at the end of the loop are spacious and shaded. The real gems are C11 and C12, situated on their own off a little loop at the south end of the campground. C11 in particular offers plenty of room under beautiful pines.

You'll find the most secluded sites for tent campers in the Twin Oaks Campground, accessed from the north side of the park's loop road. This peninsula is covered with mature oak-hickory woods and contains 31 rarely used Class D walk-in sites spread out along the 0.75 mile of road. Some are just a few steps from where you can park, while others require

Argyle Lake provides ample space for boating, fishing, or just relaxing.

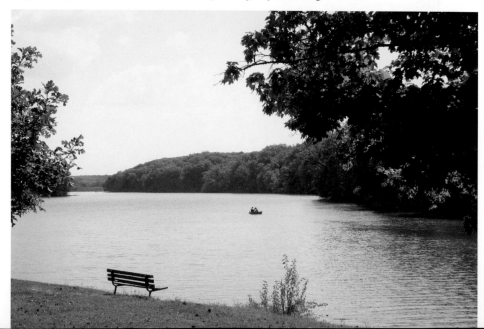

KEY INFORMATION

LOCATION: 640 Argyle Park Road, Colchester, IL 62326

CONTACT: 309-776-3422, bit.ly/ArgyleLakeIL

OPERATED BY: IDNR

OPEN: Year-round; campgrounds closed November 15–March 15

SITES: Class A: 85 sites; Class B: 23 sites; Class C: 12 sites; Class D: 31 sites

EACH SITE HAS: Picnic table, ground grill; electricity at Class A and B only

WHEELCHAIR ACCESS: Restrooms and at least one accessible tent site

ASSIGNMENT: First come, first served; reservations available online (Class A & B only)

REGISTRATION: Register with the campground host; if not available, set up and park staff will come by

AMENITIES: Water spigots, vault toilets; shower house (closed November 1– March 15)

PARKING: At site; in lot (walk-in sites)

FEE: Class A: $20/night, $30/night holidays; Class B: $18/night; Class C: $8/night; Class D: $6/night

ELEVATION: 611'

RESTRICTIONS:

PETS: On leash only

FIRES: In fire rings only

ALCOHOL: Prohibited January–May

VEHICLES: 2 per site

OTHER: 14-day limit; 1 RV and 1 tent, or 2 tents per site; 4 adults or 1 family per site

---

a hike of 0.1–0.25 mile. This area was inaccessible for several years due to the road closure, so some features haven't been well maintained. The trails to some sites are a bit overgrown, and some don't have tables or ground grills. The water spigot doesn't work, and the vault toilets noted on the park's campground map don't exist anymore, except the one on the main road at the campground entrance. Still, if you're looking for solitude, and don't mind driving to Twisted Oaks for water and showers, there are some beautiful spots here. Sites 1, 8, 9, 10, 15, 21, 24, 26, and 28 are close to the road, spacious enough and well shaded. Site 30 has a nice view of the lake. Site 31 requires a bit of a walk, since the road at the end of the peninsula is gated, but it's right on the water and well worth the extra steps.

Even if you love your own campfire cooking, plan for a meal at the park's concession, The Shanty Shack II, located on the west side of the lake. They do great breakfasts on the weekend, sandwiches and salads for lunch, and are really known for their dinner specials. Try the all-you-can-eat fried chicken on Wednesdays, fried fish on Fridays, and ribeye steaks on Saturdays, all served with salad and sides. You can eat indoors or on the covered patio overlooking the lake. The shop downstairs sells bait, ice, firewood, and snacks, and you can also rent canoes and johnboats with a trolling motor. They're open mid-April– mid-October, Wednesday–Thursday, 11 a.m.–8 p.m.; Friday–Saturday, 6 a.m.–8 p.m.; and Sunday, 6 a.m.–2 p.m. Call 309-776-3500 for more information.

Kids will enjoy the small but engaging visitor center, with hands-on exhibits, an outdoor Discovery Area, and occasional live critters on display. (A tortoise named Terra was a resident when I was last there.) Families can check out various IDNR field trip backpacks, which include guides to the natural world and tools for exploring it, like binoculars, magnifying glass, and dip net. The park naturalist also organizes special events throughout the year, including nature programs, guided hikes, and lake tours via kayak or paddleboard. Note that some activities require advance registration, and a few that use special equipment (like the kayaks) require membership in the Friends of Argyle organization for a small fee. Check the schedule at the visitor center, or under the "Interpretive" tab on the park's website for details.

Argyle Lake State Park: Twisted Oaks Campground

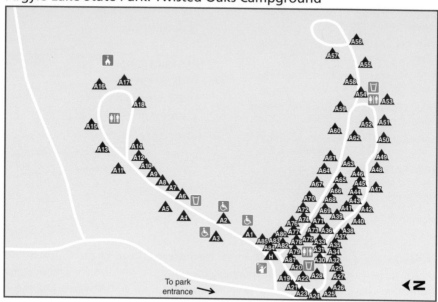

Argyle Lake State Park: Big Oaks Campground

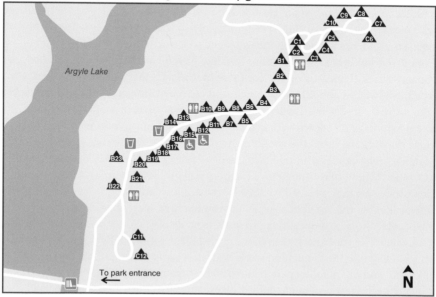

Argyle Lake State Park: Twin Oaks Campground

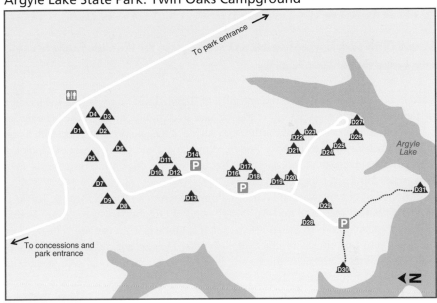

GETTING THERE

From Macomb, take US 136 about 6 miles west to Colchester. Turn right onto Coal Street and continue 1.8 miles to the park entrance on the right.

GPS COORDINATES: N40° 26.913'   W90° 48.327'

The Shanty Shack restaurant and boat rental area at Argyle Lake

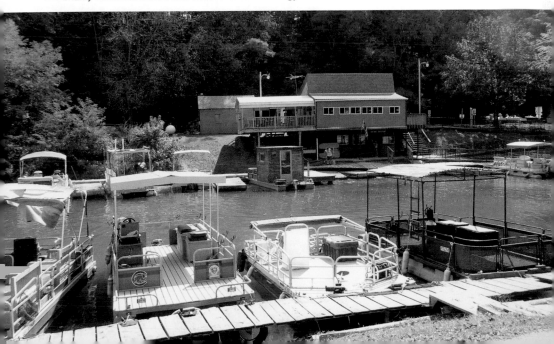

10

Beaver Dam State Park

Beauty ★★★★★ Privacy ★★★ Spaciousness ★★★ Quiet ★★★★ Security ★★★★★ Cleanliness ★★★★★

This scenic little park is a comfortable and secure place for the whole family to camp, fish, and enjoy the outdoors together.

As I drove around the bend from the entrance of Beaver Dam State Park to the lakefront, I immediately wanted to stop, get out of the car, and stretch out on one of the benches facing the lake to take in the view. The lake is the centerpiece of this picturesque park, with its gently rolling hills, mature oak and hickory woods, marshlands, and picnic areas overlooking the lake. The man-made parts—lakefront, restaurant, pavilions, docks, and restrooms—are also well maintained and attractive.

Visit on just about any weekend during camping season, and you'll see that Beaver Dam is a popular destination. From mid-April to the end of October, the campground's electric sites fill up most weekends by Friday afternoon. If solitude is what you want, Beaver Dam is probably not your first choice, at least Friday–Sunday. However, if you're looking for a comfortable, secure, and scenic place for the whole family to camp, fish, and enjoy the outdoors together, Beaver Dam is a good choice.

Beaver Dam's campground includes something for everyone. There are 66 electric sites available for RVs, and others can rough it at any of the 18 tent sites. Those who want a real bed can reserve (well in advance) the cabin right next to the modern shower house, which all campers can use. You'll all be within an easy walk of one another. Fish in the morning and teach the kids to clean their catch at the excellent fish-cleaning station by the boat launch. Rent a boat for an afternoon excursion on the 59-acre lake, or hike one of the trails around

View of the lake at Beaver Dam

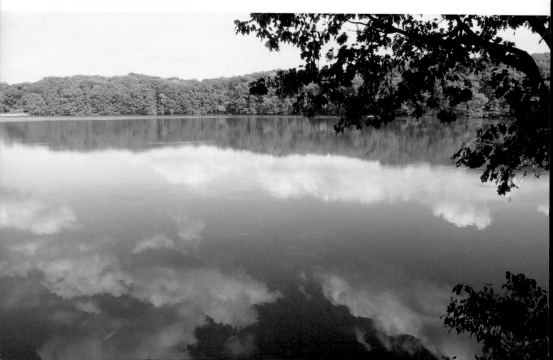

KEY INFORMATION

LOCATION: 14548 Beaver Dam Lane, Plainview, IL 62685

CONTACT: 217-854-8020, bit.ly/BeaverDamIL

OPERATED BY: IDNR

OPEN: Year-round

SITES: 66 Class A (RV) sites, 18 Class B (tent) sites, 1 cabin

EACH SITE HAS: Electricity (Class A only); picnic table, grill, and fire block; lantern pole (Class B only)

WHEELCHAIR ACCESS: Restrooms and at least one accessible electric site

ASSIGNMENT: First come, first served; reservations available online for Class A sites and cabin

REGISTRATION: Register with the campground host or at park office (if no host)

AMENITIES: Water spigots, vault toilets, shower house with flush toilets

PARKING: At campsite

FEE: Class B: $10/night; Class A: $20/night, $30/night holidays; cabin: $45/night; $5 reservation fee

ELEVATION: 608'

RESTRICTIONS:

PETS: On leash only

QUIET HOURS: 10 p.m.–7 a.m.

FIRES: In fire rings only

ALCOHOL: Not permitted

VEHICLES: 2 per site

OTHER: 14-day limit; 2 tents or 1 RV per site; 4 adults or 1 family per site

---

it. You can host the gang for supper at your campsite, equipped with two tables and plenty of space. Or you can all eat on the patio overlooking the lake at the restaurant.

As you come up the hill from the lake, the road forks, entering the campground loop. Go left and you'll enter on the RV side. During camping season, you'll find the campground host by site 1, where you can purchase firewood and register; otherwise, register at the office with staff or at the self-registration post. Most of these sites are adequate for RVs but lousy for tents. All have gravel pads and electrical hookups, with water spigots nearby, but are small and close together. Continue and you'll come to a small loop. If you must tent camp in this section, the sites on either side of the loop (15, 16, 17, 18, 24, 25, 26) are decent choices, with a bit more space and tree cover. You'll find a few more spacious RV sites if you head back to the T-intersection and turn left; these are 43, 44, and 47 on the outside of the loop.

Take the right fork from the lake (or follow the loop around from the RV side), and you'll enter the tent-camping section, with 18 sites. Most of these are refreshingly more spacious and spread out than the RV sites, though still open. All have two picnic tables, a fire block and grill, a lantern pole, and space for two vehicles. Sites 1, 2, and 3 are on a short spur, featuring some shade and a great view of the lake below. Together with sites 4–6, these sites are labeled "youth group area"; however, youth groups must reserve in advance, and if these sites are not reserved then they are open for regular camping—check with the office. Sites 7 and 8 are the most spacious and separate, and either would be my first choice. If you need two adjacent sites, some seem to be naturally paired: 9 and 10, 12 and 14, 11 and 13, and 16 and 17. All are spacious—just closer to one another. Only sites 15 and 18 are too small.

The tent and RV sites are on the same loop, but on separate ridges, with a small wooded valley between them. Forty of the electric sites and the cabin can be reserved in advance at reserveamerica.com.

Security is good here. The park is relatively small, with only a single entrance, so access is more controlled. A campground host is available around the clock in summer, and local law enforcement drive through at night. Even on weekends it's surprisingly quiet for such a popular place.

A popular spot with campers and locals at Beaver Dam has long been the Plainview Cafe at the lake, which has traditionally offered sandwiches, salads, and daily specials, and also managed boat rentals and the sale of bait, ice, and fishing supplies. At press time, management of the concession was changing hands; check with the park for current hours and details.

Beaver Dam opened in the 1890s as a private fishing club for local Carlinville businessmen, and fishing is still popular here today. The lake is stocked with largemouth bass, bluegill, sunfish, and channel catfish. Trout are restocked in the fall, and trout season opens in mid-October—expect the lake to be busy that weekend.

Beaver Dam State Park

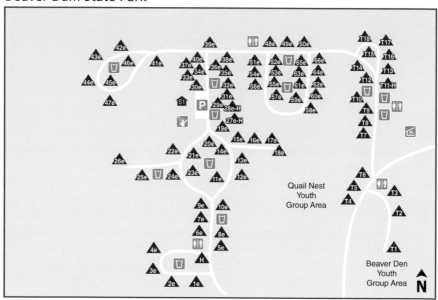

GETTING THERE

From I-55 at IL 108 (Exit 60), take IL 108 west 11 miles to Carlinville. Go through Carlinville to the Amtrak station at Alton Road. Turn left and drive 7 miles to the Beaver Dam entrance on the right.

GPS COORDINATES: N39° 12.424'   W89° 58.331'

11

⛺ COMLARA Park

Beauty ★★★★ Privacy ★★ Spaciousness ★★★ Quiet ★★★★ Security ★★★★ Cleanliness ★★★★★

COMLARA offers some excellent, serene, and even secluded spots for tent campers.

COMLARA Park is both beautiful and busy. McLean County has developed an attractive, well-maintained, and well-staffed recreational getaway here around 700-acre Evergreen Lake. The facilities are superb and the grounds manicured. Even the shower house is among the nicest I've seen in any campground. And with Bloomington–Normal's 110,000 people just to the south, it's also very popular with locals, who come to enjoy camping, boating, fishing, swimming, and trail biking. Despite this, COMLARA offers some serene and even secluded spots for tent campers in this excellent park.

Enter the park off CR 33, and stop at the visitor center on the left. If you don't have a reservation, you'll need to register here first. (After hours, you can use the self-registration post at the main campground entrance.) You can also pick up a park map and brochures on hiking, camping, or fishing, and purchase firewood and ice if you need them.

Turn right at the office and enter the campground. Yes, it's big (almost 130 sites), and probably full of RVs, but keep heading straight back. Continue past the shower house, curving left and to the back of the campground. Just past site 107 you'll reach the first of two parking areas for the 11 walk-in tent sites. The second is about 1,000 feet down the road, past site 114. The grass-covered sites are a short walk from parking, and each has a picnic table, fire ring, and scenic views of Evergreen Lake.

Walk-in campsite 8 in the White Oak area along Evergreen Lake

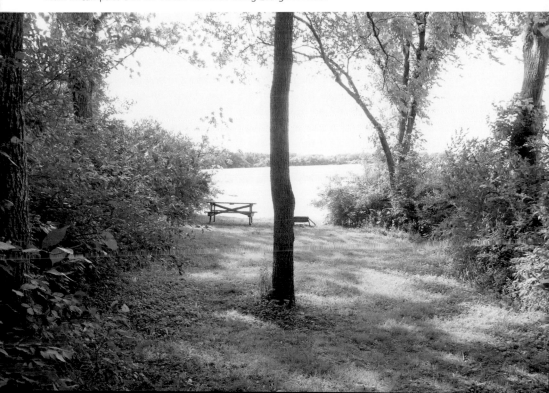

KEY INFORMATION

LOCATION: 13001 Recreation Area Drive, Hudson, IL 61748

CONTACT: 309-434-6770, bit.ly/ComlaraIL

OPERATED BY: McLean County Dept. of Parks & Recreation

OPEN: Year-round (main campground); April 1–October 15 (White Oak)

SITES: 94 electric; 23 nonelectric; 11 walk-in (main campground); 16 walk-in (White Oak)

EACH SITE HAS: Electricity (94 sites); picnic table, fire ring

WHEELCHAIR ACCESS: Restrooms and at least one accessible tent site

ASSIGNMENT: First come, first served; reservations available by phone, in person, or online at sunrisereservations.com

REGISTRATION: Register at the visitor center; at self-registration post after hours

AMENITIES: Water spigots, vault toilets, shower house

PARKING: At site, or in lot

FEE: $21/night (nonelectric), $27/night (50 amp), $24/night (30 amp); ($2 less/night for McLean County residents); $10 reservation fee online or by phone; $7 in person

ELEVATION: 746'

RESTRICTIONS:

PETS: On leash only

QUIET HOURS: 10 p.m.–8 a.m.

FIRES: In fire rings only

ALCOHOL: Not permitted

VEHICLES: 2 per site

OTHER: 14-day limit; 1 RV or 2 tents per site; no more than 8 people per site; collecting of firewood prohibited

Site 126, the first one you encounter, is beautiful and right on the lake. Surrounded by trees, it feels at least a little private, even if the rest of the campground is crowded. Sites 122, 123, and 125 are good; 124 is too small; and 118, 119, 120, and 121 are too open and close to each other. Sites 119B and 120B are my other first choices—close to the water, with trees and brush separating them from their neighbors. Since you can reserve any site at COMLARA, I recommend spending the extra $10 to hold one. Reservations can be made in person starting the first Saturday in April, and by mail or phone the following Monday.

If the main campground is too busy for you, and you don't mind walking a bit, you will love the White Oak primitive area on the other side of the lake. Go first to the visitor center to register, then head out of the park, turn left on CR 33, and turn left again on CR 8 at the stop sign. Continue 3.75 miles around the lake to the next stop sign. Turn left and go 0.75 mile to the stop sign. Park in the grassy area on the right past the stop sign, then walk past the gate and take the trail on the left to access the 16 walk-in sites. These are right on the edge of the lake, each tucked away in its own little wooded enclave, completely separate from the others. These sites are all excellent; sites 1 and 2 are closest to parking, and 14, 15, and 16 are the most isolated. To get to the farthest sites more directly, take the trail straight past the gate, pass the vault toilets, and continue across the peninsula.

Water is available back at the main campground entrance, and you can use the shower house there. The White Oak sites are open from the first Saturday in April–October 15. Surprisingly, they also book up well in advance on the weekends, so it's wise to make reservations. Even with a reservation, be sure you stop at the visitor center when you arrive—or the next morning at the latest—to get a vehicle tag.

COMLARA Park: Main Recreation Area

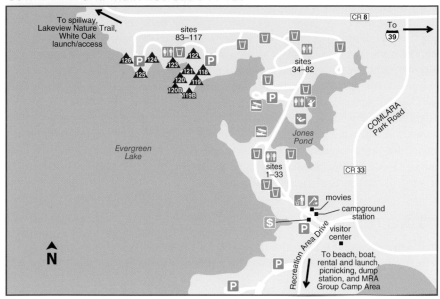

COMLARA Park: White Oak Campground

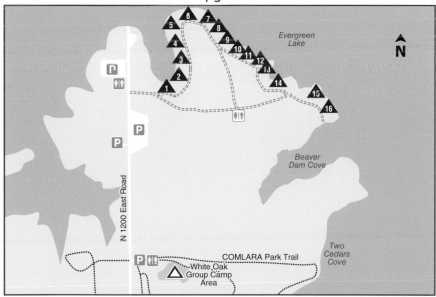

COMLARA boasts plenty of recreational opportunities, including more than 10 miles of trails for mountain biking and hiking, along with fishing, boating, and swimming. To reach the beach and main boat-launch area, turn left at the park entrance and pass the visitor center. The beachfront is actually on a separate 2.5-acre lake ringed with 4 acres of sandy beach. It features deep and shallow areas, a diving platform, a giant water umbrella, float-tube rental, showers, lockers, a playground, and a concession area. The beach is open daily from mid-May to the first Saturday in August, noon–5:30 p.m., and on weekends through Labor Day. A lifeguard is always on duty.

Right next to the beach is the boat launch. You can rent paddleboats, canoes, and row-boats with or without a motor. Check the website for rates on the beach and boat rental. If you're planning a weekend trip to COMLARA, you should also check out their events calendar. COMLARA occasionally hosts special events during the summer that may bring larger crowds, and parts of the lake may be closed.

GETTING THERE

From Bloomington, take I-39 north 8 miles to Exit 8 for CR 8. Go left (west) 1.5 miles on CR 8, then turn left on COMLARA Road (CR 33). Go 0.5 mile to the park entrance, on the left.

GPS COORDINATES: N40° 38.579'　W89° 01.782'

12

Eagle Creek State Recreation Area

Beauty ★★★★ Privacy ★★★ Spaciousness ★★★ Quiet ★★★★ Security ★★★★ Cleanliness ★★★

Lake Shelbyville has become an outdoor recreational mecca but still hasn't lost its farming-community, small-town charm.

In 1963 the U.S. Army Corps of Engineers began work in central Illinois on a dam across the Kaskaskia River, with the goal of developing a new mid-state watershed and recreational lake. The result was long, narrow Lake Shelbyville, the third-largest lake in Illinois, with 172 miles of shoreline offering a wide array of recreational opportunities.

That project has resulted in a huge lakeside leisure mecca, with hotels, restaurants, entertainment, shopping, marinas, fishing, and of course, camping. There are at least 1,500 campsites in the public and private campgrounds scattered around the lake. And, as you might expect, most cater to the RV crowd.

Despite all this development, the area still hasn't lost its farming-community, small-town charm. It's certainly not a Branson, or even a Lake of the Ozarks. Most visitors still come primarily for fishing, camping, swimming, or boating—in that order, according to a recent survey. The outdoors is still the main attraction and remains relatively unsullied by tourism.

If you'd like to enjoy Lake Shelbyville while tent camping, there are some good options. Two state parks sit across the lake from each other—Wolf Creek State Park (on the eastern shore) and Eagle Creek State Recreation Area (on the western)—and both have tent-camping areas. Choosing between the two is difficult, but Eagle Creek gets my vote, at least for camping. Eagle Creek's campground is smaller by half—smaller means fewer people. Also, Eagle

One of the spacious, wooded walk-in tent sites at Eagle Creek   *photo © Illinois Department of Natural Resources*

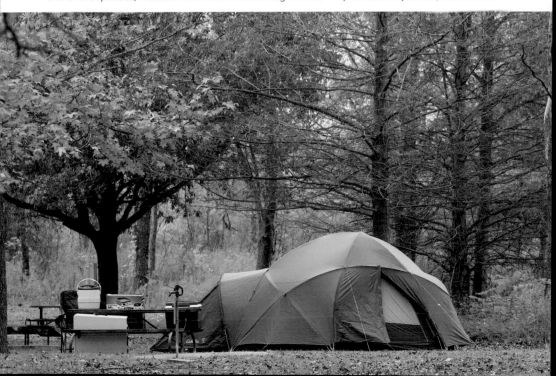

KEY INFORMATION

LOCATION: 2341 Eagle Creek Road, Findlay, IL 62534

CONTACT: 217-756-8260, bit.ly/EagleCreek-IL

OPERATED BY: IDNR

OPEN: Year-round

SITES: Class A: 148 sites; Class C: 11 walk-in tent sites, 15 drive-in tent sites

EACH SITE HAS: Picnic table, fire ring; electricity (Class A only)

WHEELCHAIR ACCESS: Restrooms and at least one accessible tent site

ASSIGNMENT: First come, first served; reservations available online (Class A only)

REGISTRATION: Set up and park staff will come by or register with the campground host

AMENITIES: Water spigots, vault toilets, shower house

PARKING: At site; at lot

FEE: Class A: $20/night, $30 on holidays; Class B drive-in: $10/night; Class C walk-in: $8/night; $5 reservation fee

ELEVATION: 663'

RESTRICTIONS:

PETS: On leash only

QUIET HOURS: 10 p.m.–7 a.m.

FIRES: In fire rings only

ALCOHOL: Permitted

VEHICLES: 2 per site

OTHER: 14-day limit; 2 tents or 1 RV per site; 4 adults or 1 family per site

---

Creek isn't generally as busy; its tent area is separate from the RV section, and the sites themselves are farther from one another.

As you enter the campground, pass the check-in station (usually unstaffed) and turn left. Proceed 0.5 mile. Make the next right, and you'll enter the parking lot for the walk-in tent sites; go straight, and you'll enter the spur for the drive-in tent sites.

Each tent section stretches along a separate, wooded ridge with plenty of shade and ends on a beautiful point overlooking the lake. In many campgrounds that have both walk-in and drive-in tent sites, the walk-ins tend to be more spacious and scenic—you get some perks for carrying your gear from the parking area. At Eagle Creek, however, I like the drive-in sites better. Of the 15 drive-in sites, 10, 12, 13, and 14 are a bit too small and close together. Site 2 is the most spacious, and site 15 is the most scenic and separate, and probably the most popular tent site on all of Lake Shelbyville.

The walk-in tent section is similarly arranged, with 11 sites. These are situated a bit more closely together and more open than the drive-in sites. The closest is just 30 feet from the parking lot, while the farthest is about 300 feet away. Again, the nicest is at the end of the point: site T11.

The tent sites are equipped with a table, a fire ring with a grill, and a lamp pole; vault toilets and water spigots are located by the entrance. A campground host will come by to register you, or you can go to the main campground to do so. Tent campers can also use the modern shower house there (closed December 1–April 1). The tent areas never fill up, and an average nonholiday weekend sees only about five sites occupied. The tent areas usually close December–April 1, mostly due to road conditions.

If you turn right at the campground check-in, you'll enter the 148-site RV section, where there are electrical hookups. If you'd prefer to camp in this area, go straight back to the dead-end loop around sites 146–148, where you'll find more space and less traffic.

While at Eagle Creek, don't miss the chance to hike along the lakeshore and admire the views. You can choose between 0.5-mile High Bluff Trail, a loop beginning near site 96 in the RV campground, and 11-mile Chief Illini Trail, which begins across the park road from the tent-camping area.

Whether you own or rent a boat, or prefer to stick to the banks, fishing is huge at Lake Shelbyville, which is home to crappie, largemouth bass, walleye, channel, and flathead catfish, bluegill, muskie, bullhead, carp, and sunfish. And for a small fee, you can swim all day at one of the four public beaches around the lake. The closest is at Wolf Creek State Park, 9 miles away. Wolf Creek Beach is open from 10 a.m.–sunset, and costs $1 per person, and the three beaches operated by the U.S. Army Corps of Engineers open at 8 a.m. and cost $5 per vehicle. Beaches and pools are usually open from Memorial Day to Labor Day, but that may be affected by water levels, so call or check online first.

If you want to keep busy, the Lake Shelbyville area boasts a wide range of other attractions, from golf courses, bike trails, and wineries, to a monument to the local woman who invented the automatic dishwasher. See lakeshelbyville.com and bit.ly/USACE-Shelbyville to scope out your options.

Eagle Creek State Recreation Area: Tent Campground

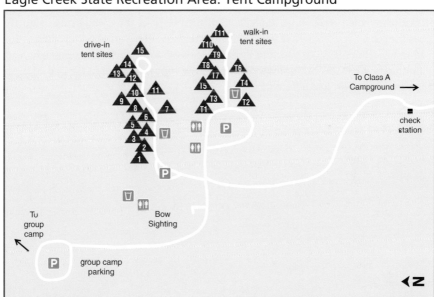

GETTING THERE

From Decatur, take IL 121 south to IL 128 in Dalton City. Turn right, go 14 miles south to Findlay Road (CR 2100 North), and turn left. Drive 4 miles to the Eagle Creek sign (CR 2200 East), and turn right. Head 0.75 mile, turn left at the sign, and go 1 mile to the park entrance.

GPS COORDINATES: N39° 30.595'   W88° 43.149'

13

⚑ Forest Glen Preserve

Beauty ★★★★ Privacy ★★★ Spaciousness ★★★ Quiet ★★★★ Security ★★★★★ Cleanliness ★★★★★

Don't miss the stunning view of the Vermilion River valley from the top of the 72-foot-tall observation tower.

I knew that Forest Glen Preserve was another underappreciated gem when a staff member told me they often get visitors from Danville—14 miles away—who are surprised to discover this beautiful spot virtually in their own backyard. Forest Glen is a surprise. On the drive there, you'd swear there's nothing but cornfields, until you stumble across this enclave of 1,800 acres of wooded ravines and tall-grass prairie adjacent to the Vermilion River. The well-maintained grounds, facilities, and hiking trails, along with a variety of interpretive programs, make it easy to enjoy this diverse bit of west-central Illinois.

Forest Glen also does tent camping right—there's a separate campground for tent campers that's walk-in only and is just far enough from parking to keep vehicle noise to a minimum but not too far to carry your gear. And all campers get to use the showers in the main campground—pretty much ideal for me.

As you enter the preserve, go straight, then turn right at the campground sign. You'll first pass the ranger station, where you'll return to register after you've set up camp—they're open Monday–Thursday, 5–6 p.m. and Friday–Sunday, noon–8 p.m. The next right leads to the walk-in tent area. You can unload your vehicle in the circular lot at the end of the road and then park in the lot just before it.

The Vermilion River valley stretches beneath you from the deck of the observation tower at Forest Glen.

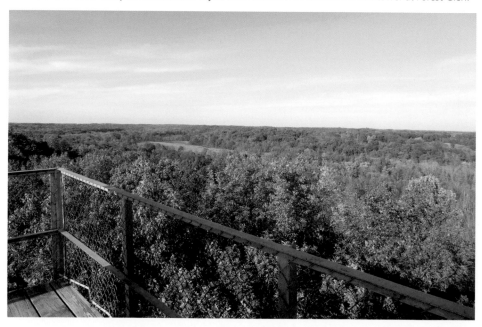

KEY INFORMATION

LOCATION: 20301 East 900 North Road, Westville, IL 61883

CONTACT: 217-662-2142, vccd.org/giforestglen.html

OPERATED BY: Vermilion County Conservation District

OPEN: Year-round

SITES: 14 walk-in tent sites, 34 electric sites, 8 nonelectric sites, 2 backpacking areas

EACH SITE HAS: Picnic table, fire ring

WHEELCHAIR ACCESS: Restrooms and at least one accessible electric site

ASSIGNMENT: First come, first served

REGISTRATION: Set up first, then register at ranger station; backpackers must register in advance

AMENITIES: Water spigots, vault toilets, shower house

PARKING: In lot (walk-in sites); at site

FEE: Nonelectric & walk-in sites: $17/night; electric sites: $22/night; backpacking sites: $10

ELEVATION: 640'

RESTRICTIONS:

PETS: On leash only

QUIET HOURS: 10 p.m.–8 a.m.

FIRES: In fire rings only

ALCOHOL: Permitted

VEHICLES: 2 per site

OTHER: 14-day limit; 1 RV and 1 tent, or 2 tents per site; no collecting of firewood

---

The walk-in tent-camping area consists of a loop with 14 sites, all wooded and well shaded, each with a table and fire ring. Generally, the sites on the outside of the loop are larger and farther apart, and most look out over the wooded ravine and small creek that encircles this little hill. Sites 1, 2, 5, 7, and 13 are a bit small, but sites 3, 4, 6, and 12 are more spacious. Sites 8, 9, 10, and 11 are clustered together—any one of these would be fine if the others weren't occupied. Site 14 is my first choice—it's set apart from the others yet still close to parking. No site is far, though—you won't walk more than 200 feet to get to any of them. There is a water spigot and some vault toilets beside the loop entrance. On an average fair-weather weekend, you can expect this campground to be half full.

Instead of turning right toward the walk-in campground, continue straight and you'll end up at the family campground. These 42 sites all have gravel pull-ins, a table, and a large fire ring, and they offer plenty of grass-covered space for pitching a tent. Pass the campground host and shower house and turn right to reach the eight nonelectric sites on the south side of the road—29, 30, 33, 34, 37, 38, 41, and 42. These are large sites, though not as well shaded as those in the walk-in campground. Willow Creek Pond sits behind them, and there's a small fishing dock by site 33. The campground host also sells firewood and ice.

Backpackers can camp for $10 at one of two places along the 11-mile River Ridge loop trail, at the 3-mile and 7.5-mile points. You must register in advance, preferably at least a week. The registration form is available on the website and can be emailed or faxed in. The trail begins at the staff office parking lot. Detailed trail maps are available at the office or online.

If you have a head for heights and your legs can stand the climb, you shouldn't miss the view from the top of the 72-foot observation tower. As you enter the park, take the second right, following the signs to the observation-tower parking. The hike is 0.2 mile down a wide gravel path along a ridge with wooded valleys on either side. Most old fire towers around the state have either been torn down or locked up over liability concerns, but this one is open sunrise–sunset, and each level is reassuringly surrounded by chain-link fence. (You should still hang on to smaller children when ascending.) Enjoy the stunning view of the Vermilion River valley before descending to hike 0.15 mile down to the Vermilion itself. Here you can connect with other well-marked trails, ranging from easy to rugged. Pick up a trail guide and map at the staff office.

On weekends Forest Glen offers a variety of activities that families with kids will particularly appreciate. North of the campgrounds, check out the Sycamore Hollow Nature Center, open on Sundays 1–4 p.m. from Memorial Day to Labor Day. Here you can see mounted birds and mammals, touch pelts, examine rocks and arrowheads, and learn from the interpretive displays. Also on Sunday afternoons, head up the hill to see living history reenacted at the Pioneer Homestead. The first Saturday of the month from June through October, join your camping neighbors for a free one-hour hayride. Meet at the staff office: June–August at 7 p.m., and September and October at 6 p.m. Check the website and staff office for a schedule of guided hikes and other special activities.

GETTING THERE

From I-74, take Exit 215 and follow Georgetown Road (US 150) south 4.2 miles. Turn left on Main Street at the CVS pharmacy and follow the road 7.3 miles to the park entrance, on the left.

GPS COORDINATES: N40° 00.003'   W87° 33.327'

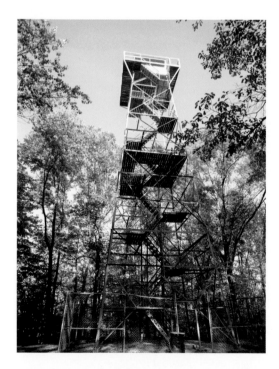

The observation tower at Forest Glen is open sunrise–sunset.

Forest Glen Preserve Family Campground

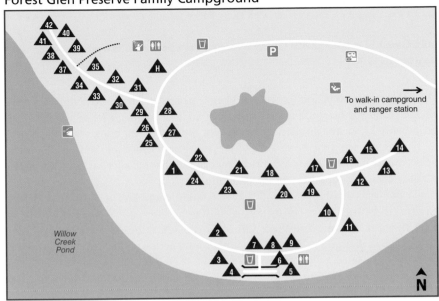

Forest Glen Preserve Walk-in Tent Campground

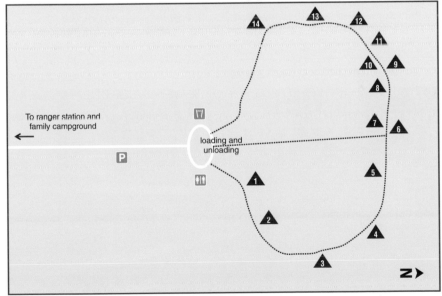

14

⚘ Friends Creek Conservation Area

Beauty ★★★★ Privacy ★★★ Spaciousness ★★★ Quiet ★★★★ Security ★★★★★ Cleanliness ★★★★★

Friends Creek is a quiet park and campground that celebrates the prairies of central Illinois.

Folks who are not from Illinois (or who are from Chicago, which almost counts as a separate state) often think Illinois south of I-80 consists of nothing but mile after mile of flat corn and soybean fields. I hope the diversity of landscapes covered in this book serves to dispel that myth. However, around my hometown of Decatur in the center of the state, it's true. The glaciers scraped us smooth and left a rich layer of soil that defaults to luxurious prairie or, with a little coercion, supports vibrant agriculture.

Amid the fields and farms, Friends Creek Conservation Area is a park that celebrates the prairie. There are mature oak-hickory woods, to be sure, and its namesake creek winds through the area, but much of these 526 acres consists of beautiful open meadows and restored tallgrass prairie. The clean, quiet campground here is popular with locals but hardly known outside the area.

The campground consists of one large loop, with an avenue running down the middle. Most of the 26 electric sites are along the central road and west (left side as you enter); the 9 nonelectric sites are around the outer loop east. In addition to everything being clean and beautifully maintained (as are all the properties in the Macon County Conservation District), the sites are spacious, and many of the nonelectric ones are canopied by tall, spreading oaks. The sites on the outside of the loop to the right as you enter—26, 29, 31, and 33—are my first choices for that reason. If you want electricity, I recommend site 25,

Take a hike on the Sunshine Trail at Friends Creek.

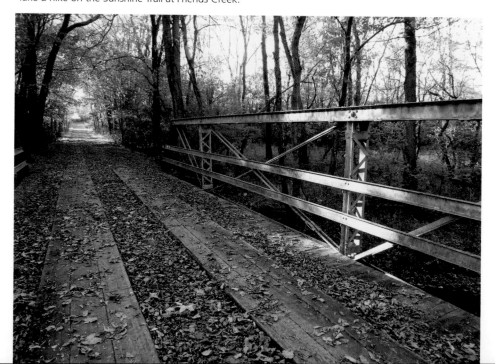

KEY INFORMATION

LOCATION: 13734 Friends Creek Park Road, Cisco, IL 61830

CONTACT: 217-423-7708, bit.ly/FriendsCreekIL

OPERATED BY: Macon County Conservation District

OPEN: May 1–October 31

SITES: 9 nonelectric, 26 electric

EACH SITE HAS: Picnic table, fire ring

WHEELCHAIR ACCESS: Restrooms and at least one accessible tent site

ASSIGNMENT: First come, first served; reservations available by phone with credit card

REGISTRATION: Register with the campground host or at the self-registration board

AMENITIES: Water spigots, vault toilets, shower house

PARKING: At site

FEE: Nonelectric: $10/night for Macon County residents ($12/night for nonresidents); electric: $17/night for county residents ($20/night for nonresidents); $5 reservation fee

ELEVATION: 679'

RESTRICTIONS:

PETS: On leash only

QUIET HOURS: 10 p.m.–6 a.m.

FIRES: In fire rings only

ALCOHOL: Not permitted

VEHICLES: 2 per site

OTHER: 14-day limit; 1 RV or 2 tents per site; 6 people per site

---

tucked into the trees at the southeast corner, or site 21. Those at the back are along a fence with farmland on the other side and aren't as attractive. You'll find water spigots throughout the campground and an excellent shower building in the center. You can register with the campground host (at site 1) or at the self-registration board at the shower house.

You won't come to Friends Creek for solitude. On most weekends, all of the electric sites will be occupied by RVs, probably reserved well in advance. This is one of the few campgrounds I'm recommending where you might camp across the road from a trailer. However, the regulars who come to Friends Creek are a quiet bunch. You can usually walk in and get a good nonelectric site, or you can reserve one in advance by credit card.

You can explore more of the woods and prairie around Friends Creek if you cross the highway to the parking area by the historic Bethel School. From there you can access two loop trails. As the name implies, the 2-mile Woodland Trail traverses woods before heading along Friends Creek. Sun Trail makes a 2.5-mile circuit through woods and across a gently sloping hillside meadow.

You can fish, but not swim, in Friends Creek. There is a superb 1,000-foot beach about 10 miles north at Clinton Lake, if you feel like taking a dip. It's usually busy on warm days, but there's plenty of room to spread out, and there are also changing rooms and showers. The large swimming area is marked by buoys and ranges from wading-pool shallow (for the little ones) to about 6 feet deep. The concession at the southern end sells sandwiches, snacks, and drinks. The beach is open from Memorial Day to Labor Day, from 10 a.m.–7 p.m., and the cost is $2 per person. Call 217-935-8722 for more information. From Friends Creek, turn right out of the park onto Friends Creek Park Road and head 9.25 miles north until you cross the lake. Then take the first left into Clinton Lake State Park and follow the road and signs down to the beach.

If you want to do something more than lie in a hammock in the shade (although that is a fine way to spend the day at Friends Creek), my favorite local place to hike is the Rock Springs Conservation Area, about 30 minutes away on the southwestern edge of Decatur. This is another Macon County Conservation District property, with 1,343 acres of woods and prairie. Here you can hike up some actual hills (albeit small ones) along the 9 miles of interconnected trails that traverse the area. From the visitor center, you can also hop on the paved 7-mile bike trail that extends to the north side of Decatur. My favorite hike is the 2.5-mile River Trail that follows the Sangamon River (the lower portions may be flooded or muddy in the spring). Trail maps are available at Friends Creek. Don't miss the nature center, which has live fish and reptiles, a bird-watching window, and excellent interactive exhibits that kids will enjoy. To get to Rock Springs from Friends Creek, take I-72 west toward Decatur to Exit 133, which puts you on US 36 East. Go to the stoplight and turn right onto Wyckles Road. Drive 2.1 miles to Rock Springs Road, turn left, go 1 mile to Brozio Lane, and then head 0.5 mile to the entrance, on the left.

Friends Creek Conservation Area Campground

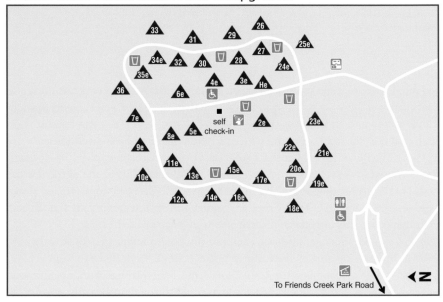

GETTING THERE

From I-72 at Exit 156, go north 0.7 mile on IL 48 to Duroc Road. Turn left and go 1 mile to Friends Creek Park Road. Turn right and drive 0.25 mile to the park entrance, on the right.

GPS COORDINATES: N40° 01.793'   W88° 47.008'

15

Jim Edgar Panther Creek State Fish and Wildlife Area

Beauty ★★★★ Privacy ★★★ Spaciousness ★★★★ Quiet ★★★★ Security ★★★★★ Cleanliness ★★★★★

Camp in one of the unique three-sided wooden shelters and enjoy central Illinois's longest mountain-biking trail.

Jim Edgar Panther Creek State Fish and Wildlife Area (JEPC) is one of Illinois's newest parks, and everything about it sparkles. The campgrounds are immaculate, the buildings clean and modern, and the trails well maintained. And JEPC is *big*—16,550 acres of rolling terrain—offering a beautiful mix of woods, prairie, lakes, and ponds, plenty to do, and camping options from the luxurious to the comfortably primitive.

Because JEPC covers such a huge area, there are various entrances, but the main one is from Ashland or Petersburg off Newmansville Road to the east. Go 1.4 miles from this entrance west to the office, turn left, and proceed less than 1 mile south to the main Prairie Lake Campground on the left. Stop here first to register with the campground host, where you can also purchase ice and firewood.

Go south from the main campground entrance to Wolf Road, where you'll see a sign for group and primitive camping. Turn left, then right, and go 0.2 mile to the walk-in camping parking lot. There are seven walk-in sites, spread along a well-mown grass trail, on the

View from the shores of Prairie Lake

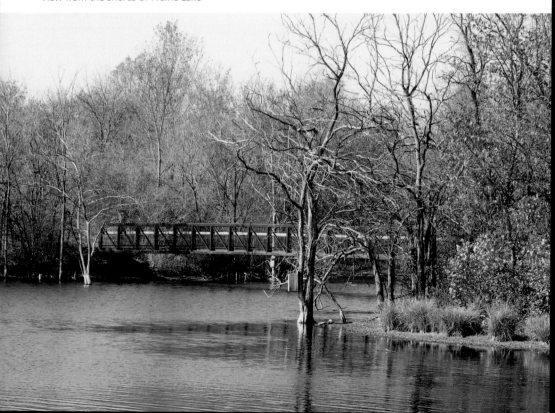

KEY INFORMATION

LOCATION: 10149 CR 11,
Chandlerville, IL 62627

CONTACT: 217-452-7741, bit.ly/JimEdgarIL

OPERATED BY: IDNR

OPEN: Year-round

SITES: Class A: 64 electric; Class AA: 18 full-hookups; Class D: 7 walk-in; 9 cabins

EACH SITE HAS: Electricity (Class A & AA);
sewer and water (Class AA); Picnic table,
fire ring; wooden shelter (Class D)

WHEELCHAIR ACCESS: Restrooms and at
least one accessible electric site

ASSIGNMENT: First come, first served; cabins
and group campground reservable online

REGISTRATION: Register with the
campground host

AMENITIES: Water spigots, vault toilets,
shower house

PARKING: At site (Class A & AA); in lot
(Class D)

FEE: Class A: $20/night, $30/night holidays
(add $5 for Class AA); Class D: $6/night/
tent (add $2/night for shower use); cabin:
$45/night

ELEVATION: 599'

RESTRICTIONS:

PETS: On leash only

QUIET HOURS: 10 p.m.–7 a.m.

FIRES: In fire rings only

ALCOHOL: Not permitted

VEHICLES: 2 per site

---

edge of the woods to the north. They're about 100–200 feet apart, and because of the way the trail curves you're mostly out of sight of your neighbors. Chances are you won't have many—this area doesn't always fill up, even on holiday weekends, and on an average fair-weather weekend only two or three sites will be occupied.

Each site is equipped with a fire ring, table, trashcan, and, unique to JEPC in Illinois, a three-sided, roofed wooden shelter. Like everything else at JEPC, these look brand-new, sturdy, and attractive. They're about 10 feet deep and provide protection from rain and sun, large enough that I've seen some campers simply stretch a tarp across the entrance and camp inside. My favorite is site 5—it's the most secluded, tucked back into the woods—but the main criterion for choosing is how far you're willing to walk, from 0.1 mile for site 1 to less than 0.5 mile for site 7. The trail is smooth, and a wagon works well to transport your gear to the site. The vault toilets are located opposite site 3. You will need to get water at the group or main campground and can use the main shower house.

Either of the two group campgrounds, if not already taken or reserved, is available to individuals and family groups. They don't offer much shade, but there's lots of open space for pitching tents, plus water, restrooms, and a picnic shelter with electricity. Your "group" may be small, but you'll have to pay for a minimum of 10 people. You can reserve one of these online for an additional $5.

The main campground doesn't offer much shade either, but it is pretty, with spacious, flat, front-lawn kind of grassy expanses. All sites have electricity, but with a tent you'll want to avoid the expense of the 18 full-hookup sites. If you do want a bit of luxury, reserve one of the nine cabins well in advance. Each has two bunk beds, a double bed, a table, a ceiling fan, a heater, and electricity. You'll need to bring your own bedding. All are right on the lake, but cabins 8 and 9 are more secluded, with woods around.

JEPC offers plenty of recreational opportunities. Many come to fish, either in the 210-acre Prairie Lake (stocked with muskie, along with the usual panfish and catfish) or in one

Jim Edgar Panther Creek SFWA: Prairie Lake Campground

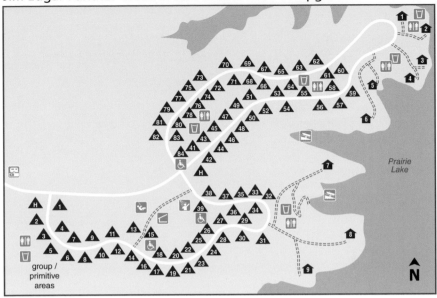

Jim Edgar Panther Creek SFWA: Walk-in Tent Area

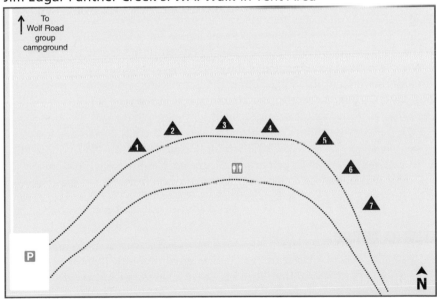

of the smaller, less busy lakes or ponds. Cyclists can enjoy the 9-mile paved biking loop trail, or the 24 miles of mountain-biking trail in two loops. With the gentle terrain at JEPC, the latter is fairly tame but scenic. It's open to bikers from April 16–October 31, and only to hikers during the rest of the year. For equestrians there is a 51-site campground and 26 miles of trails.

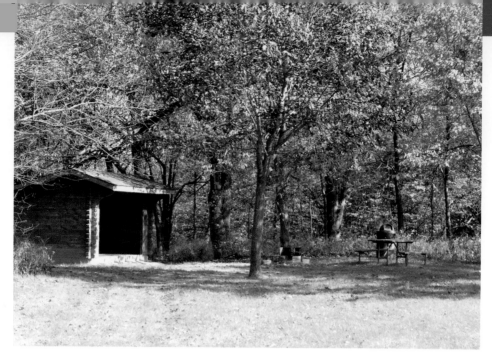

One of the attractive wooden camping shelters at Jim Edgar Panther Creek

There are no facilities for renting canoes or boats at JEPC, but you can bring your own. Trolling motor and canoe access are allowed at Gridley and Drake Lakes, and Prairie Lake has unlimited horsepower with a no-wake zone for the entire lake.

If you enjoy history, do not miss New Salem State Historic Site, south of nearby Petersburg. New Salem is a reconstruction of the village where Abraham Lincoln spent his early adulthood. You can tour the village homes, shops, museum, and visitor center; view demonstrations of daily life and work in the 1830s; and take in plays and concerts in the 250-seat outdoor theater. If you want to squeeze a bit of education into the kids' vacation, download any of the free activity guides available on the website. There is no admission cost, only a suggested donation. Call 217-632-4000 or visit lincolnsnewsalem.com for more information. To get there from JEPC, go north 0.25 mile on Newmansville Road, follow it as it curves right and continues 11 miles into Petersburg (and becomes Douglas Street). Turn right on IL 123/97, and go 2.3 miles south to New Salem.

GETTING THERE

From Springfield, take I-72 west to Exit 76, then go north on IL 123. Go 11 miles to the T-intersection at IL 125 in Ashland. Turn left, go 2.8 miles to Newmansville Road, and turn right at the brown JEPC sign. Go 7 miles to the JEPC entrance on the left.

GPS COORDINATES: N39° 59.986'   W90° 02.562'

16

Kickapoo State Recreation Area

Beauty ★★★★ Privacy ★★★ Spaciousness ★★★ Quiet ★★★★ Security ★★★★ Cleanliness ★★★★

Come to Kickapoo for the chance to canoe Illinois's only National Scenic River.

Kickapoo State Recreation Area is a great place to play. Sure, the campsites are spacious, tent campers can use the shower house, and there's a terrific little restaurant—but the prime attraction is recreation. The park offers scenic (and even rugged) hiking and mountain biking, excellent fishing, scuba diving, and the opportunity to canoe Illinois's only National Scenic River. You could come here for a quiet, do-nothing weekend—but why?

Kickapoo owes its diverse recreation and terrain to the fact that these lands were once open strip mines. The state of Illinois purchased them in 1939, and over the years nature has transformed them into deep, clear ponds, steep hills, and wooded ravines. Twenty-two ponds and lakes cover more than 220 of Kickapoo's 2,842 acres, providing ample space for lots to do.

As you enter the park from the east, go about 0.25 mile past the bridge to the entrance to Brian Plawer Campground on the right. If someone is on duty at the check-in station, register there; otherwise, set up at an unreserved site and return later. Take the first right past the check-in station and go down the hill to the Erie loop of the campground. As you enter the loop, you'll see the sign for the Sauk tent-camping area on the left. On the right is the grassy clearing where you can park after you've unloaded your gear.

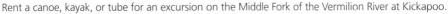

Rent a canoe, kayak, or tube for an excursion on the Middle Fork of the Vermilion River at Kickapoo.

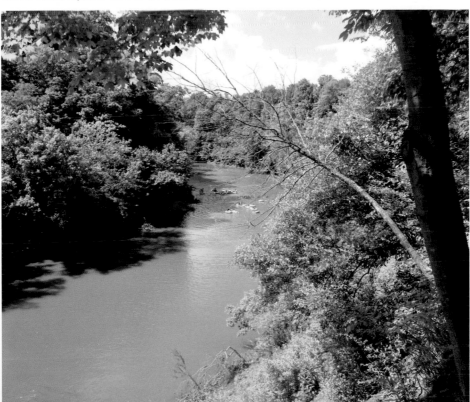

KEY INFORMATION

LOCATION: 10906 Kickapoo Park Road, Oakwood, IL 61858

CONTACT: 217-442-4915, bit.ly/KickapooIL

OPERATED BY: IDNR

OPEN: Year-round

SITES: Class A: 100 electric sites;
Class B: 64 nonelectric sites;
Class C: 18 walk-in tent sites

EACH SITE HAS: Electricity (Class A only);
picnic table, fire ring

WHEELCHAIR ACCESS: Restrooms and at least one accessible electric site

ASSIGNMENT: First come, first served

REGISTRATION: Set up first, then register at the office

AMENITIES: Water spigots, vault toilets, showers (may be closed in winter)

PARKING: At site (Class A & B); in lot (Class C)

FEE: Class A: $20/night, $30/night holidays;
Class B: $10/night; Class C: $8/night; $2 less when showers are closed

ELEVATION: 559'

RESTRICTIONS:

PETS: On leash only

QUIET HOURS: 10 p.m.–7 a.m.

FIRES: In fire rings only

ALCOHOL: Permitted

VEHICLES: 2 per site

OTHER: 14-day limit; 1 RV and 1 tent, or 2 tents per site; 4 adults or 1 family per site

---

The 18 walk-in tent sites, numbers 102–119 (in reverse order from the parking lot) extend along a 0.25-mile footpath that parallels a ridge overlooking the lake below. All are sufficiently spacious, with a picnic table and ground grill. Vault toilets are behind site 110, and water spigots are available in the campground loops at either end of the tent area. There isn't much brush between you and your neighbors, but sites 106 and 109 are set back the farthest from the trail and offer the most space. On an average nonholiday weekend, this area is about half full, so you should be able to find something suitable.

Besides the walk-in sites, many of the drive-in sites are surprisingly large, with plenty of flat grassy space for pitching tents. If you'd prefer a drive-in site, it's generally best to go for one of the smaller loops, such as Fox, with 15 electric sites, or Erie, with 33 nonelectric sites, and try for those on the outside of the loop. In Erie, if you need two adjacent sites, I recommend 132 and 133, 148 and 149, or 150 and 152. For a single site, I really like 129, which is spacious and right by the stairs down to the large fishing dock on Long Lake. In Fox, site 90 is nice; 95 is my favorite, with a beautiful view of the lake below. Most of these can also be reserved in advance for an additional $5 at reserveamerica.com.

The Illini and Miami loops of the campground offer more-typical RV sites and would be my last choice for tent camping. If you are stuck there, try for sites 74–81 on the east side of Illini—they're a bit bigger and back up to woods. Kickapoo has a secondary campground—Redear Campground—0.5 mile south of the intersection past the bridge at the park entrance. It has 30 nonelectric sites, water, and vault toilets, and campers can use the showers in Plawer Campground. I don't think its sites are nearly as attractive as the good sites in the main campground.

In my opinion, Kickapoo can also boast one of the nicest, friendliest, and best-run park concessions in Illinois. Kickapoo Adventures is located just past the bridge into the park. They offer 8- or 13-mile canoe or kayak trips and shorter tube trips on the Middle Fork of the Vermilion River, or you can rent a canoe, kayak, or stand-up paddleboard by the hour, half day, or day to explore Clear Lake and Inland Sea in the park. The best part is that for some trips they shuttle you upstream and you head back to their office—no need to wait for or hurry to meet a bus at your takeout point. You can even check your keys at the boathouse, so you don't risk losing them in the river. They also offer canoe lessons, mountain bike rentals, and guided bike trips, and sell bait, fishing supplies, ice, firewood, and snacks. Check kickapooadventures.com for current information and to reserve rentals (recommended particularly on weekends).

Next to Kickapoo Adventures is the Park Bistro, open daily for lunch and dinner from Memorial Day to Labor Day (breakfast on Saturday and Sunday), and on the weekends in the fall and spring. You can enjoy live music there on selected evenings during the spring and summer. Call 217-446-6986 or check their page at facebook.com/kickapooStatePark for more information.

Kickapoo is one of the few parks in Illinois that allows scuba diving. If you register and show proper certification, you can dive in Sportsman's Lake or Inland Sea. Don't expect crystal-clear waters—visibility is usually 10 feet or less—but it's worth trying if you enjoy diving.

There are also more than 13 miles of singletrack, directional mountain-biking trails of varying degrees of difficulty in the park. The local Kickapoo Mountain Bike Club maintains these trails, and you can find trail maps and descriptions, as well as recent conditions, on their website, kickapoomountainbike.org.

Kickapoo State Recreation Area Campground

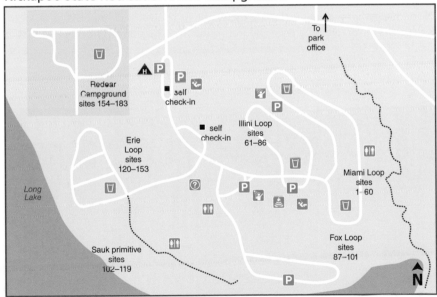

GETTING THERE

From I-74, take Exit 206 north onto Newtown Road. Go 1 mile, turn right at the park sign onto CR 1880 North, then go 2 miles to the park entrance.

GPS COORDINATES: N40° 08.249' W87° 44.890'

17

⛺ Lincoln Trail State Park

Beauty ★★★★ Privacy ★★ Spaciousness ★★★ Quiet ★★★★ Security ★★★★★ Cleanliness ★★★★★

Hike among the smooth gray beech trees, which have changed little since the days when the Lincolns passed this way.

Illinois is known as the Land of Lincoln, and many sites around the state commemorate events from the life of the state's most famous resident to reach the White House. Fifty years after Lincoln's death, the state decided to mark the exact route traveled by Lincoln's family when they moved from Kentucky to Illinois. Eventually the 1,000-mile Lincoln Trail was established, and the state park of the same name lies just west of the trail as it follows Illinois Route 1.

Lincoln Trail State Park covers more than 1,000 acres of densely wooded hills and ravines around a U-shaped 146-acre lake. It's a beautiful destination for hiking, boating, and fishing, and offers two very different campgrounds with some scenic tent-camping spots. Add some luxuries like an excellent shower house and a great restaurant, and it's worth spending a relaxing weekend here.

As you enter, turn left on the loop road that encircles the lake to head toward the camp-grounds. The first entrance on the left is for the impeccable but aptly named Plainview Campground. Plainview has 129 sites neatly arranged in open grassy sections. Everything is well manicured and clean, including the excellent shower building. But your view will be of the rows of surrounding RVs, and the young trees have not yet come into their own for shade. Most sites are electric, except for the Class B sites on the far east side of the

Welcome to some of the best walk-in tent sites in Lakeside Campground.

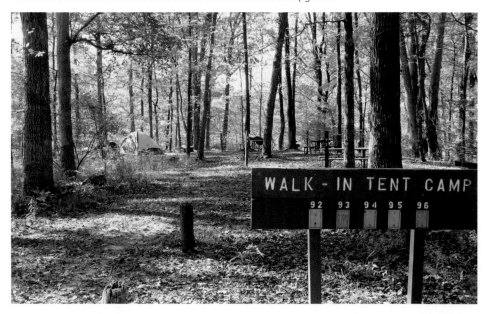

LOCATION: 16985 East 1350th Road, Marshall, IL 62441

CONTACT: 217-826-2222, bit.ly/LincolnTrailIL

OPERATED BY: IDNR

OPEN: Year-round

SITES: Class A: 190 electric sites; Class B: 11 nonelectric sites; Class C: 27 walk-in tent sites

EACH SITE HAS: Picnic table, fire ring and grate; electricity at Class A only

WHEELCHAIR ACCESS: Restrooms and at least one accessible tent site

ASSIGNMENT: First come, first served; reservations available online for most sites

REGISTRATION: Register with the campground host; if not available, staff will come by

AMENITIES: Water spigots, vault toilets, shower house

PARKING: At site (Class A & B); in lot (Class C)

FEE: Class A: $20/night, $30/night holidays; Class B: $10/night; Class C: $8/night; $5 reservation fee

ELEVATION: 633'

RESTRICTIONS:

PETS: On leash only

QUIET HOURS: 10 p.m.–7 a.m.

FIRES: In fire rings only

ALCOHOL: Permitted

VEHICLES: 2 per site

OTHER: 14-day limit; 1 RV and 1 tent, or 2 tents per site; 4 adults or 1 family per site

campground: 55, 57, 59, 61, 63, 65, 66, 84, 85, 87, and 89. If you want an electric site here, try for one of the pull-through sites 2–12 (even)—which offer the most shade and space.

Lincoln Trail's second campground, Lakeside, is just down the road on the right, and it's starkly different. Here you'll find plenty of mature woods and, appropriately enough, some great views of the lake that surrounds it on three sides. Most of the 99 sites have electrical hookups and pull-in gravel pads, but 26 walk-in tent-only sites are scattered among them in small pockets. The tent sites are 30–33, 61–74, 84–87, and 92–96. Each is a short walk from the adjacent parking area and has a table, ground grill, and lantern pole. All are on the lake, but my favorites are 84–87, which have nice flat tent pads, and 61–65, which have towering trees for shade. If you need two sites, grab 73 and 74, and you'll have the spot all to yourselves. If you want electricity, I recommend site 13, which is beautiful, overlooking a ravine, and is right by the entrance to Beech Tree Trail, or else sites 45, 46, or 88–91, which are right on the lake. There are water spigots and vault toilets throughout, and all campers can use the showers in Plainview (open year-round). The sites in the tent areas are a bit close together and might feel crowded on a really busy weekend, but this campground almost never fills up, least of all the walk-in sites. If you want to be sure of getting a preferred site, most can also be reserved online for an additional $5 at reserveamerica.com.

Behind site 14 in Lakeside Campground, you can pick up the scenic 0.5-mile Beech Tree Trail, which proceeds along wooden stairways and bridges and down to the lake. Along the way you'll skirt the American Beech Woods Nature Preserve, passing among the smooth gray beech trees that have changed little from the days when the Lincolns passed this way. The reward at the end is the excellent and popular Lincoln Trail Family Restaurant, which features dinners, sandwiches, a salad bar, ice cream, and specials. It's open April–October: Monday–Friday, 10:30 a.m.–8 p.m.; Saturday, 8 a.m.–8 p.m.; and Sunday, 8 a.m.–2 p.m. (closed Mondays in the fall). Their Sunday breakfast buffet is popular with campers and locals alike. Even if you do all your own campfire cooking, the view of the lake from the restaurant makes it worth coming in just for pie and coffee. For more information, call 217-826-8831 or check their Facebook page (facebook.com/LincolnTrailRestaurant).

Downstairs from the restaurant are the marina and bait shop; here you can purchase fishing supplies, snacks, ice, and firewood, and rent rowboats, paddleboats, hydrobikes, and fishing boats with trolling motors. Fishing is good, and the 7 miles of wooded shoreline are well worth exploring.

If you want more hiking, try the 2-mile Sand Ford Nature Trail in the southwest corner of the park, or the brand new 3.1-mile Air Strip Trail on the north side. You can get even more of a workout on the 8-mile trail system at Fox Ridge State Park, about 30 miles to the west. The camping there is best left to RVs, but the hiking is rigorous, scenic, and well worth the side trip. Fox Ridge consists of a series of ravines along a glacial moraine, so the trails include lots of ups and downs, with many wooden stairs and bridges to help. If you go there, be sure to scale the 144 steps to the Eagle's Nest deck, overlooking the Embarras (pronounced "ambraw") River. Fox Ridge is about 6 miles south of Charleston on IL 130.

Lincoln Trail State Park: Lakeside Campground

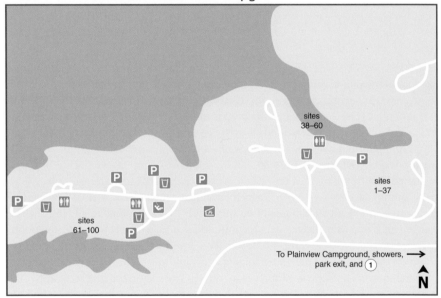

GETTING THERE

From I-70, take Exit 147 at Marshall to IL 1. Go 5.2 miles south to CR 1350 North. Turn right and drive 1 mile to the park entrance.

GPS COORDINATES: N39° 20.805'   W87° 42.207'

18

Lodge Park

Beauty ★★★ Privacy ★★★★ Spaciousness ★★★★★ Quiet ★★★★ Security ★★★★ Cleanliness ★★★★

Camp beside the rippling waters of the Sangamon at a site perhaps hundreds of yards from neighbors.

I have hiked and camped all over Illinois and have lived within 30 miles of Lodge Park for half of my life. I've even worked occasionally at Allerton Park, just 8 miles away. Yet until I began researching this book, I didn't know this little gem of a campground existed.

According to the ranger at this Piatt County Forest Preserve, most people don't. Lodge Park encompasses only about 500 acres straddling the Sangamon River. It doesn't have a website or offer a brochure or even a campground map. Visitors who stumble across it are often just as pleasantly surprised as I was. Lodge Park offers the chance to camp right beside the rippling waters of the Sangamon at a site perhaps hundreds of yards from the nearest neighbor. You can do a little fishing and hiking, but you'll come here for a tranquil stay with few neighbors, leaving you with fields, woods, and water almost to yourself.

The ranger will tell you Lodge Park offers "roughly 15" campsites. The uncertainty is due to the fact that much of the campground is open field, and campers can set up anywhere within that area. The more or less official sites, unnumbered, are wherever you see a picnic table and fire ring—I counted 13. The camping area consists of a large loop, about 1.5 miles around, with a single road bisecting the loop from the entrance.

The fishing pond at Lodge Park

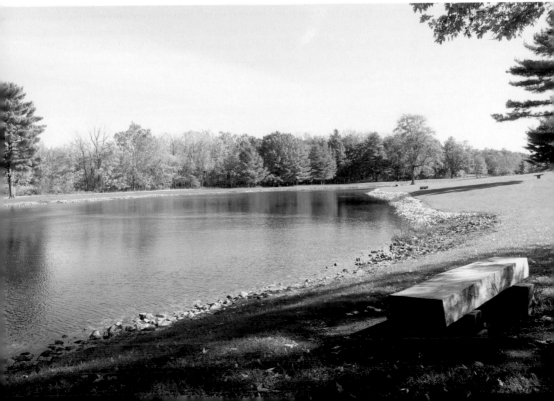

KEY INFORMATION

LOCATION: 1852 North Old Route 47,
Monticello, IL 61856

CONTACT: 217-762-4531, bit.ly/LodgeParkIL

OPERATED BY: Piatt County Forest
Preserve District

OPEN: Year-round (but closed to vehicles
December 1–April 1)

SITES: About 13

EACH SITE HAS: Picnic table, grill, fire ring

WHEELCHAIR ACCESS: Not designated

ASSIGNMENT: First come, first served

REGISTRATION: Set up and park staff will
come by

AMENITIES: Water spigots, vault toilets

PARKING: At campsite or off road nearby

FEE: $10/night

ELEVATION: 663'

RESTRICTIONS:

PETS: On leash only

QUIET HOURS: 10 p.m.–6 a.m.

FIRES: In fire rings only

ALCOHOL: Not permitted

VEHICLES: 2 per site

OTHER: 14-day limit; 3 tents, or 1 RV and
1 tent per site

Drive around the southern part of the loop, and you'll find other sites scattered in a grassy field, some with large trees, and most close to water and restrooms. Those south of the road across are spacious but closer together; those just north of it are farther apart. For the best site in this area, take the entrance road straight across the field and turn right. Away from the road, this site affords a great view of the Sangamon and has some wooded cover.

The star campsites for privacy are the four in the mixed pine and deciduous forest at the northern end. For these you'll have to park roadside and walk a bit, at most 100 feet. The reward is a sense of isolation rarely found at any established campground.

Head north, counterclockwise around the loop, and watch for a trail into the woods. This will lead you to the first wooded site, hidden from the road. The next, at the northernmost point, is right on the Sangamon River. It was muddy when I visited because it had recently rained; it can flood when the river is high. The next two, in the northwest corner of the campground, are my favorites. The one on the east is larger and overlooks the river, while the one to the west is well away from the road—watch for the trail, or you'll drive right past it.

Reservations are not accepted, but Lodge Park is rarely full, even on Memorial Day or Labor Day weekends. The only exception is around July Fourth, when the park is packed with campers and is the site of Monticello's fireworks display. Don't come looking for peace and quiet from about June 20 to July 5! Occasionally, scout or youth groups camp here as well, but they usually give notice, so you can call ahead to see if you'd be sharing the grounds with a large group.

Lodge Park is open for camping year-round. However, it is closed to vehicular traffic December 1–April 1. You can park at the entrance and walk in, but you'll have to carry your gear. Also, note that the park is down the road from a small subdivision, so you may see some locals jogging or walking dogs.

When water levels are low enough (usually in the summer), you can also cross the Sangamon on foot via the concrete ford in the southwest corner of the campground. There are about 150 wooded acres with clearly marked trails on the other side. If you don't mind getting your feet wet, you can sometimes camp over there—check with the ranger for permission.

From Lodge Park you can also visit nearby Allerton Park, voted one of the "seven wonders of Illinois" by state residents. Allerton was the estate of the gentleman farmer and art collector Robert Allerton, who devoted three decades to developing the ornamental gardens surrounding his manor house. Today the University of Illinois manages the park for recreation, education, and research purposes. You can hike more than 14 miles of well-marked trails through the gardens, unique statuary, and natural areas adjacent to the Sangamon River.

Allerton is open 8 a.m.–sunset. The manor house itself now serves as a conference center and is usually not open to the public. For trail maps and more information, stop by the visitor center, or visit allerton.illinois.edu. To get there from Lodge Park: Take I-72 west to Exit 164, then turn left onto Bridge Street. Drive 0.5 mile, turn right onto Old SR 47, and go 2 miles to CR 625 East. Turn left, go 1 mile to the T-intersection, turn right, and drive 0.5 mile to the entrance to Allerton, on the left.

Lodge Park Campground

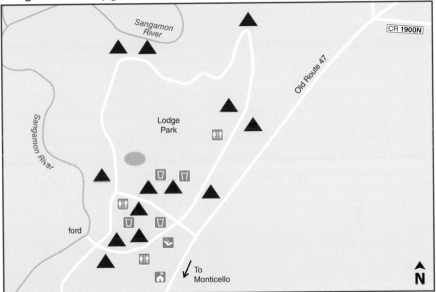

GETTING THERE

From Decatur, take I-72 East to Exit 166, turn right, then make the next right onto Old Route 47. Drive 0.5 mile north to the park entrance, on the left.

From Champaign, take I-72 West to Exit 169 and turn right onto Old Route 47. Go 2.5 miles south to the park entrance, on the right.

GPS COORDINATES: N40° 03.771'   W88° 33.751'

19

⚑ McCully Heritage Project

Beauty ★★★★ Privacy ★★★★★ Spaciousness ★★★★ Quiet ★★★★★ Security ★★★★ Cleanliness ★★★★

You'll probably have this little camping area all to yourself.

Calhoun County in western Illinois is almost an island—35 miles long and barely 6 miles wide for most of its length, it's a hilly, heavily wooded peninsula tucked between the Illinois and Mississippi Rivers. To get there from the east, west, or south requires using the single bridge or one of three ferries. Visitors can discover small towns, secluded wild places, and even archaeological excavations that reveal 8,000 years of human habitation. And amid all of this is one quiet place to tent camp: the McCully Heritage Project.

McCully is a private nonprofit foundation, the legacy of Howard and Eva McCully, established to promote environmental education and enjoyment of the natural, cultural, and historical resources of the lower Illinois River valley. Today the foundation manages these 940 acres for a variety of programs, including limited primitive camping.

I have described some campgrounds as "underappreciated" or "less frequented"— McCully could be called "virtually unknown," at least in terms of camping. The campsites are never full, and on many weekends you may have the area all to yourself.

When you arrive at McCully, park in the lot in front of the pavilion. Walk left, past the white house that serves as the office and visitor center, and behind the office you'll see a signboard directing you to the campsites. Put your donation in one of the envelopes and slip it into the red box.

The five campsites are situated northwest of the barn and surrounded by woods. Some are more shaded, and all are spacious enough for several tents. You'll find a picnic table and fire ring, and probably some firewood neatly stacked there for your use—if not, help

View of the Illinois River valley from the southern trails at the McCully Heritage Project
photo by Michelle Berg Vogel/McCully Heritage Project

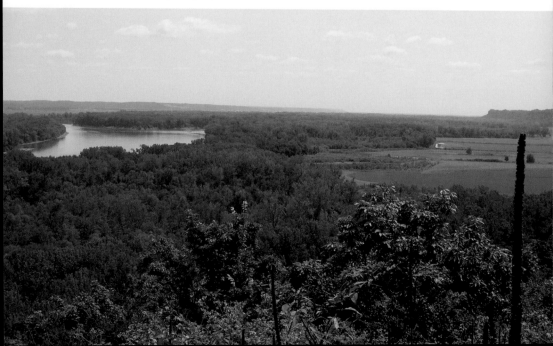

KEY INFORMATION

LOCATION: 592 Crawford Creek Hollow Road, Kampsville, IL 62053

CONTACT: 618-653-4687, mccullyheritage.org

OPERATED BY: McCully Heritage Foundation

OPEN: Year-round

SITES: 5 primitive walk-in sites, 2 hike-in sites

EACH SITE HAS: Picnic table and fire ring (walk-in sites only)

WHEELCHAIR ACCESS: Restrooms

ASSIGNMENT: First come, first served

REGISTRATION: Register at the self-registration kiosk

AMENITIES: Water spigots, restrooms, shower house

PARKING: At lot

FEE: $10/night suggested donation; $5 donation requested for firewood

ELEVATION: 457'

RESTRICTIONS:

PETS: On leash only

QUIET HOURS: Unspecified, but be respectful of other campers

FIRES: In fire rings only

ALCOHOL: Not permitted

VEHICLES: 2 per site

OTHER: No cutting or gathering of firewood

---

yourself to the pile under the pine tree behind the barn, and leave a donation in the box. Restrooms with flush toilets and showers are by the sign-in board (two of the four are fully accessible), and water pumps there and by the barn. There's nothing spectacular in terms of scenery or even isolation—you're still fairly close to the road and the house where the groundskeeper lives—just simple campsites, and probably no one else camping. Though it's not required, I suggest calling ahead if you want to camp—there's always the possibility a school group has scheduled a field trip the very day you want to come.

McCully's 940 acres offer plenty of places to explore. Go north past the campsites to see the historic 19th-century log cabin. Just beyond that are two ponds where you can fish or just watch turtles sunning themselves. South of the road is a boardwalk trail through a wetland. Beyond this is about 15 miles of secluded hiking trails, mostly wooded, with abundant wildlife and scenic overlooks of the Illinois River valley. You will have to work a bit to enjoy it—the entrance to McCully lies in a valley, and everything to the north and south is uphill. But the rewards are well worth it. You may see some of the myriad bird species that have been sighted there, as well as deer, wild turkey, fox, coyote, and even the elusive bobcat. From the southernmost overlook, you can see 21 miles downriver to Pere Marquette State Park. The 12 miles of trails to the south are the most extensive, and a trail map is necessary—you'll find copies at the information kiosk and online. Note that the southern trails may be shared with equestrians April 15–October 1.

For backpackers, there are also two hike-in campsites in the southern section, each less than 1 mile (uphill!) from the wetland parking area. There are no facilities, just a clearing in the woods, but it's certainly peaceful. Or you can rent a rustic house with electricity, water, and vehicular access. Call for more information.

If you think archeology means pyramids and ancient Egypt, check out the Center for American Archeology in Kampsville, on IL 100 just south of the ferry crossing. This fascinating museum focuses on the prehistory of the area around the confluence of the Illinois and Mississippi Rivers, which has been called the "Nile of North America" for the sophisticated

American Indian settlements that developed there as far back as 6000 BC. The museum is open from late April through the Sunday before Thanksgiving, Tuesday to Sunday. Admission is free, but donations are appreciated. Check their website, caa-archeology.org, or call 618-653-4316 for information on special programs.

McCully is just 25 miles north of the much better known (and much busier) Pere Marquette State Park, popular for its scenic trails and rustic Civilian Conservation Corps–built lodge. However, that campground is often busy—so camp at McCully, drive down for the day, and have dinner in the excellent lodge dining room. To get there, take IL 100 south almost 25 miles to the park entrance, on the left. For more information on area attractions, check greatriverroad.com.

McCully Heritage Project Campground

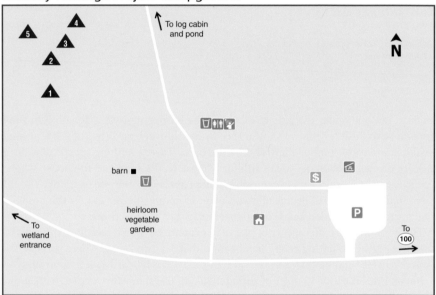

GETTING THERE

Follow IL 108 west to the Illinois River (54 miles from I-55, Exit 60; 22 miles from US 67). Take the free ferry (which runs 24 hours) across the river to Kampsville, then turn left onto IL 100. Go 1.1 miles south to Crawford Creek Road, turn right, and go 0.5 mile to the entrance, on the right.

GPS COORDINATES: N39° 16.938'   W90° 37.298'

20

Moraine View State Recreation Area

Beauty ★★★★ Privacy ★★★★★ Spaciousness ★★★ Quiet ★★★★ Security ★★★★ Cleanliness ★★★★

The prime attraction of the 10 Tall Timber campsites is their seclusion from one another.

At Moraine View State Recreation Area, you can view something very old and something very new. Approaching the park from the south, you'll see a long high rampart running east to west. The park sits atop this end moraine, a ridge of earth and rock that was left behind by the glaciers as they retreated north at the end of the last Ice Age, some 20,000 years ago.

Once you get atop the moraine, scan the horizon to the north and east, and you'll be able to see some of the 240 white wind turbine generators of the Twin Groves Wind Farm.

Besides the geology and technology, Moraine View offers some good camping options, as well as fishing, hiking, swimming, and boating. While the 137-site Gander Bay RV campground fills up virtually every weekend during camping season, the walk-in campgrounds are a better choice for tent campers and not as busy.

If you want to park close to your campsite and don't mind the possibility of having neighbors, choose among the 22 walk-in sites at the Catfish Bay Tent area. Sites 21 and 22 are closest to parking (less than 100 feet away), and those farthest (sites 11 and 12) require a hike of only about 350 feet. Catfish Bay is on a small hill, is moderately shaded, and overlooks the lake. The sites are somewhat open to one another, and the ground slopes toward the water in places. Each site has a table and ground grill; you'll find water and the vault toilets in the parking lot. Sites 1 and 2 are wheelchair accessible and are only open to other campers if unoccupied after 8 p.m., and then only for one night. If you want space and no slope, site 3 is great. If you prefer a bit more distance and foliage between you and the neighbors, sites 16 and 18 are good. I like camping by the water's edge, so sites 9 and 11 are my first choices.

Explore the lake at Moraine View in a rental kayak, or bring your own.

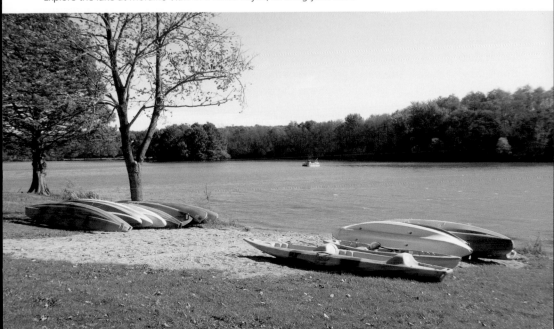

KEY INFORMATION

LOCATION: 27374 Moraine View Park Road, LeRoy, IL 61752

CONTACT: 309-724-8032, bit.ly/MoraineViewIL

OPERATED BY: IDNR

OPEN: Year-round

SITES: Class A: 137 RV sites and 30 equestrian sites; Class D: 22 walk-in and 10 backpacking sites

EACH SITE HAS: Electricity in Class A only; picnic table, grill, fire block

WHEELCHAIR ACCESS: Restrooms and at least one accessible electric site

ASSIGNMENT: First come, first served; reservations available online for 102 Class A sites

REGISTRATION: Register with campground host (Class A); self-registration (Class D)

AMENITIES: Water spigots, vault toilets; shower house (Class A only, closed November 1–mid-April)

PARKING: At campsite (Class A); at trailhead (Class D)

FEE: Class D: $6/night; Class A: $20/night, $30/night on holidays; $5 reservation fee

ELEVATION: 851'

RESTRICTIONS:

PETS: On leash only

QUIET HOURS: 10 p.m.–7 a.m.

FIRES: In fire rings only

ALCOHOL: Not permitted

VEHICLES: 2 per site

OTHER: 14-day limit

Unfortunately, even these walk-in sites will be full on a holiday weekend; they can even fill up on regular weekends during good weather. They're not reservable, so plan to arrive early.

If you prefer more solitude and don't mind hiking a bit, check out the Tall Timber backpacking area. The prime attraction of these 10 sites, shaded by mature hardwoods, is their seclusion from one another. These sites are the last to go on a busy weekend, and even if they're all occupied, you won't see your neighbors. Laid out in a 1.5-mile loop in the woods, each site has a table and a fire ring. The longest hike in this area is to site 6 (about 0.5 mile), but the other sites are much closer. Start at the parking lot, where the self-registration signboard will show you which sites are open. Go right (counterclockwise) around the loop, and you'll reach site 1 in about 800 feet. And if you have more gear than you want to lug even that distance, you can pull off to the side of the road closest to site 1 (you'll see the picnic table through the woods), carry everything to the site, and then go park at the trailhead. The only disadvantage to site 1 is its proximity to the road—it's a little harder to imagine yourself alone in the wilderness with the sound of the occasional car going by.

All of the Tall Timber sites offer plenty of space and shade, but my favorite is site 10, both because it's not a long walk (less than 1,000 feet) and because it's a little different from the others. From the parking area, hike straight ahead (south) about 250 feet until you see the first side trail to the left. This junction isn't well marked, so you'll have to watch for it. Turn left and head east and southeast about 700 feet. Site 10 is perched above the banks of Salt Creek and is close enough to the end of the lake that you can just hear the water tumbling over the dam. If this is music to your ears, this spot's perfect for you.

Moraine View Restaurant & Kayak Rental, near the boat dock, is open daily; offers canoe, kayak, and boat rentals; and sells tackle, bait, snacks, and some supplies. The restaurant serves breakfast and lunch, and you can eat on the patio overlooking the lake or take your meal back to your campsite. Check their website (moraineview.com) for rental rates and menus. Though the walk-in tent sites don't include access to the shower house at Gander Bay, for $2 per day ($3 on weekends and holidays) you can take advantage of the beach, open most days from Memorial Day to Labor Day, 10 a.m.–6 p.m.

Moraine View State Recreation Area Campgrounds

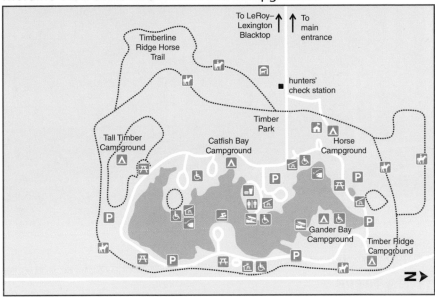

Tall Timber Backpacking Tent Sites

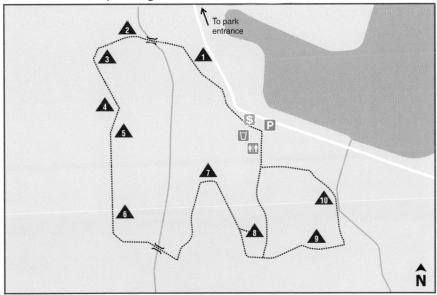

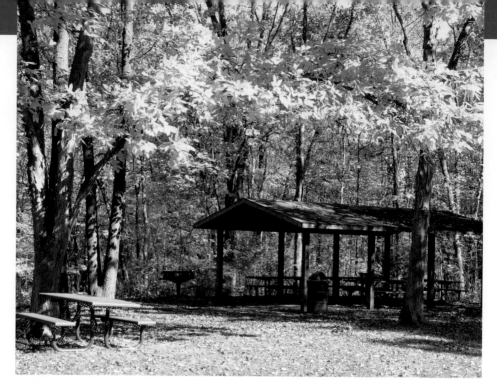

Moraine View has beautiful spots for picnicking.

GETTING THERE

From I-74 at Exit 149, head 0.5 mile north to US 150 in LeRoy. Turn left. Continue 0.6 mile to West Street (CR 21). Turn right, and go 4.1 miles north to park sign on the right.

GPS COORDINATES: N40° 24.803'   W88° 43.608'

21

⚠ Ramsey Lake State Recreation Area

Beauty ★★★★ Privacy ★★★ Spaciousness ★★★★ Quiet ★★★★ Security ★★★★★ Cleanliness ★★★★★

Ramsey Lake is a fisherman's park, and multiple campgrounds offer some nice, quiet choices for tent campers.

Ramsey Lake State Recreation Area features 1,980 acres of wooded hills and valleys, with its beautiful 46-acre namesake lake as the centerpiece. Most people come here for the lake—fishing and boating are popular, and camping is almost as popular. There are multiple campgrounds, though, and most campers gravitate to the one best suited for RVs, leaving some nice quiet choices for tent campers.

First, the best choice. From the park entrance, take the first right and go north to the fork and left at the Pine Bend Campground sign. Because it is small—just six walk-in sites—this secluded area can occasionally fill up on weekends. But if it's not completely full, the sites are spacious enough that you'll have plenty of privacy—and midweek you could easily have it all to yourself. The two sites south of the loop are just 25 feet from parking and spread beneath two massive oaks. If you want to get farther from any casual traffic that might drive through to explore, settle at one of the four sites on the north side. The farthest is a 225-foot walk and has the best tree cover. All have a ground grill and table. Vault toilets are by the road, but you'll need to get water at one of the other campgrounds.

Ramsey Lake is a scenic fishing paradise.

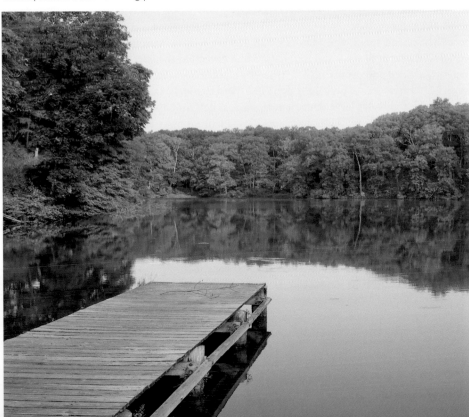

KEY INFORMATION

LOCATION: Ramsey Lake Road, Ramsey, IL 62080

CONTACT: 618-423-2215, bit.ly/RamseyLakeIL

OPERATED BY: IDNR

OPEN: Year-round (White Oak); other campgrounds closed at least December–March

SITES: Class A: 90 sites (White Oak); Class B: 24 group sites; Class C: 38 sites (Hickory Grove); Class D: 6 walk-in sites (Pine Bend); 1 cabin

EACH SITE HAS: Picnic table, grill; electricity (Class A & B only)

WHEELCHAIR ACCESS: Restrooms and at least one accessible electric site

ASSIGNMENT: First come, first served; reservations available online (Class A only)

REGISTRATION: Register at the office or with the campground host

AMENITIES: Water spigots, vault toilets, shower house (closed December 1–April 1)

PARKING: At site (Class A, B, C); in lot (Class D)

FEE: White Oak: $20/night, $30/night holidays; group: $18/night; Hickory Grove: $8/night; Pine Bend: $6/night; cabin: $45/night

ELEVATION: 619'

RESTRICTIONS:

PETS: On leash only

QUIET HOURS: 10 p.m.–7 a.m.

FIRES: In fire rings only

ALCOHOL: Permitted

VEHICLES: 2 per site

OTHER: 14-day limit; 1 RV or tent or 2 smaller tents per site; 4 adults or 1 family of 6 per site

---

The second-best choice for tent camping is Hickory Grove Campground, with approximately 38 drive-in sites (my count—the park website says 45). From the park entrance, take the first right, then make a left and go past the group campground. Sites 112–130 are in the grass along the roadside, and you can park on the grass. Those on the right (112–120) have more shade and space, and 118, 119, and 120 are well away from the road. I like site 112, which is the farthest back and has mature tree cover. On the left, 121, 122, and 123 are sufficiently shaded and roomy; 127–130 are, by comparison, cramped. Farther down the road, sites 9–111 have gravel pull-ins. I don't like these as much, except for 110, at the end of the loop to the right—it's large, and right by vault toilets and a small playground. All the sites have a ground grill and table, and most have a lantern pole. Hickory Grove is rarely more than half full, so you should be able to find a suitable site most weekends.

A third possibility is the group campground you pass on the way to Hickory Grove. These 24 sites are set up in groups of three and have tables, ground grills, and electricity, plus a big fire ring for each group. They're open to individual campers if not already taken or reserved by a group. Sites 22–24 are the best choice here—farthest from the road, with lots of room to spread out under the trees. They are reservable for $5 more per site; you must reserve a minimum of six sites.

White Oak is the Class A campground, with 90 electric sites, a shower house (closed December 1–April 1), and a rental cabin with beds, electricity, heating, and air-conditioning. From the park entrance, go straight to White Oak Campground on the right. This would be my last choice for tent camping, but it's the only option from around December 1–April 1 (depending on weather), when the other campgrounds are closed. Whichever site you settle on, be sure to register at the park office (8 a.m.–4 p.m.) or after hours with the campground host in White Oak (site 41, by the showers) before setting up. Note that all campers can use the shower house except those in the Class B group area (a quirk of the IDNR's site classification system). You can reserve some White Oaks sites and the cabin through reserveamerica .com for an additional $5.

Ramsey Lake is a fisherman's park, and the lake is stocked with largemouth bass, bluegill, redear, channel catfish, and black crappie. There are five floating docks—off White Oak, Hickory Grove, and the youth group campgrounds—from which you can fish. The concession at the lake sells bait, ice, and firewood, but there is no longer any boat rental.

For hikers, there's a 1.8-mile loop trail, with trailhead parking by the office. Equestrians will find a small horse campground 1 mile north of the main park entrance, linked to a 15-mile loop that explores the terrain away from the lake.

Do take time for a slow drive on the scenic and hilly 4-mile loop around the lake (one-way clockwise). At the less visited rear section of the park, perched on ridges overlooking the lake, you'll find some nice picnic areas where you might be tempted to spend a few solitary hours enjoying the view, reading a book, or taking a nap.

Ramsey Lake State Recreation Area Campgrounds

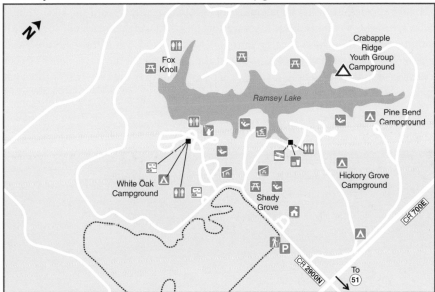

GETTING THERE

On IL 51, go 15 miles south of Pana, or 13 miles north of the intersection of IL 51 and I-70 in Vandalia. Turn west onto CR 2900 at the brown park sign, then go 1 mile to the park entrance.

GPS COORDINATES: N39° 09.567'   W89° 07.310'

22

Sam Parr State Fish and Wildlife Area

Beauty ★★★★ Privacy ★★★ Spaciousness ★★★★ Quiet ★★★★ Security ★★★★ Cleanliness ★★★★★

The walk-in tent sites on the lakeshore are well worth the short hike.

When I was a kid, I never understood how my great-grandfather could sit fishing for hours, even with nothing biting. I realize now that fishing was just an excuse to enjoy the outdoors, and whether the fish cooperated or not was immaterial. I'm reminded of that because Sam Parr State Fish and Wildlife Area is just a few miles from where my great-grandfather lived most of his life and is just the sort of peaceful place he loved. The terrain is typical of central Illinois—a mix of low timbered hills and prairie, with a narrow V-shaped 183-acre lake at the center. The park doesn't have a lot of amenities, but the separate tent-camping area offers quiet lakeside camping and a good place to enjoy fishing, boating, and simply relaxing.

As you enter Sam Parr off IL 33, go 0.3 mile, to the second road on the right, and follow the signs for tent camping. The walk-in tent area is at the southwest corner of the lake and has 21 sites spread out over a large grassy lawn sloping gently toward the lake. Though all the sites are visible to one another, most are spacious and widely separated. Some are close to parking, so you don't have to carry your gear very far at all, while those on the lakeshore require a short hike of 300–450 feet. Most of the time you should have plenty of choices. The walk-in area is busy on holidays, but other weekends may only see two or three parties camping, and it's rarely even half full.

Many of the walk-in campsites at Sam Parr sit right on the lake.

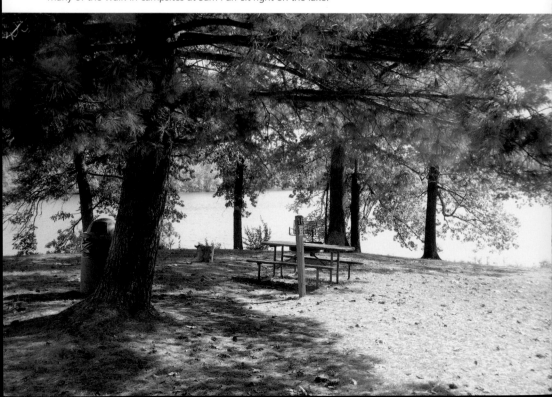

KEY INFORMATION

LOCATION: 13225 East IL 33,
Newton, IL 62448

CONTACT: 618-783-2661, bit.ly/SamParr-IL

OPERATED BY: IDNR

OPEN: Year-round

SITES: Class B/E: 33 electric sites;
Class D: 21 walk-in tent sites

EACH SITE HAS: Picnic table, fire ring or
ground grill; electricity in Class B/E only

WHEELCHAIR ACCESS: Restrooms and at
least one accessible tent site

ASSIGNMENT: First come, first served

REGISTRATION: Select site, then register
at the office

AMENITIES: Water spigots, vault toilets

PARKING: At site (Class B/E); in lot (Class D)

FEE: Class B/E: $18/night; Class D: $6/night

ELEVATION: 523'

RESTRICTIONS:

PETS: On leash only

QUIET HOURS: 10 p.m.–7 a.m.

FIRES: In fire rings only

ALCOHOL: Permitted

VEHICLES: 2 per site

OTHER: 14-day limit; 1 RV and 1 tent,
or 2 tents per site; 4 adults or 1 family
per site

Site 1 is attractive but too close to the parking lot for my comfort—you'll see and hear everyone who drives in. If you want to be close to your vehicle, try sites 2, 3, 11, or 14, which are a bit farther away and shaded by pine or maple trees. I prefer the sites on the fringes (out of the line of foot traffic) and closest to the lake. Sites 6, 8, 9, 10, 16, and 20 all fit the bill. Site 8 is on a bit of a slope but is pretty and well shaded. My two favorites are site 9—not much shade but a beautiful view of the lake, and right by a little fishing dock—and site 20. They're the farthest from parking but well worth the extra steps. Most nonholiday weekends you'll have few if any neighbors in this area.

Each site has a table and a fire ring or a ground grill; vault toilets and a water spigot are located near the parking lot. Only the water spigot at the park office is open in winter. Once you've selected a site, register at the office if it's open, on the first road to the right as you enter the park. Otherwise, just set up, and staff will come by the next day.

The RV campground, with 33 electric sites, is at the end of the park road, to the north and around the lake. The location is beautiful—a wooded peninsula between the arms of the lake—but the sites are small, with gravel pads and not a lot of tent space. On most fair-weather weekends this campground will be busy to full.

Sam Parr has 2 miles of foot trails, and the nicest section, along the lakeshore, begins at the dam on the southern end. There are two boat ramps, but no boat rental or concession.

If you enjoy natural history, check out Prairie Ridge State Natural Area, about 10 miles southwest of Sam Parr. These 4,100 acres of tall prairie and marsh are the last refuge of the once-abundant prairie chicken and home to numerous other state endangered or threatened species. From late March–April, you may be privileged to witness the loud "booming" of the male prairie chicken's courtship dance. Limited access means roadside viewing, except around the office and in the portion owned by the Illinois Audubon Society. To get to the Prairie Ridge office from Sam Parr, take IL 33 for 2.5 miles into Newton, then turn left onto Liberty Street (1100 East). Drive 3.8 miles south to 600 North, turn right, go 1 mile west to 1000 East, turn left, and travel 1.75 miles south to the white house with the wire fence. The Robert Ridgway Nature Preserve of the Audubon Society, with trails and an observation deck, is located 0.25 mile farther south, then 0.6 mile east. For more information, see bit.ly/ILAudubonRidgeway.

For more conventional history, visit the Lincoln Log Cabin State Historic Site, 30 miles north of Sam Parr. The site includes a replica of the log cabin in which Abe Lincoln's father and stepmother lived when they moved to Illinois in 1837, as well as a working period farm. Costumed site interpreters present pioneer life, and on a given day you may witness shearing sheep, carding wool, harvesting wheat, making brooms, or maybe even the visit of an itinerant 19th-century physician. The site is open daily except for holidays, from 9 a.m.– 5 p.m. Living history programs of various sorts take place between May 1 and October 31. From Sam Parr, head 23.5 miles north on IL 130 to 1200 North—watch for a "Lincoln Cabin" sign. Turn left, go 4 miles west to 1450 East, then turn right and follow the road 2.6 miles north to the main entrance. Check lincolnlogcabin.org for more information.

Sam Parr State Fish and Wildlife Area: Tent Campground

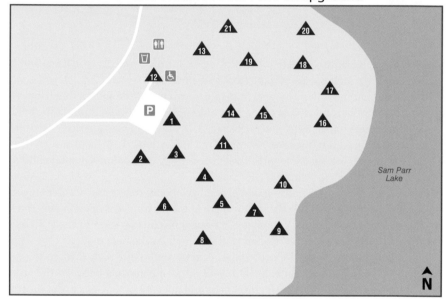

GETTING THERE

From I-70 at Greenup, take Exit 119 and drive 17 miles south on IL 130 to IL 33. Turn left and go 0.75 mile to the park entrance, on the left.

GPS COORDINATES: N39° 00.750'   W88° 07.602'

23

Sand Ridge State Forest

Beauty ★★★★ Privacy ★★★★★ Spaciousness ★★★ Quiet ★★★★★ Security ★★★★ Cleanliness ★★★★★

Explore miles of forest trails in Illinois's desert, complete with prickly pear cactus.

For a state presumed to be all cornfield, Illinois boasts an amazing diversity of habitat: wetlands and forests, bluffs and meadows, canyons, and a wealth of lakes and rivers. One expanse of wilderness southwest of Peoria is even reminiscent of the desert. Sand Ridge State Forest sits atop 7,500 acres of sandy soil, about half oak-hickory forest, one-third pine, and much of the rest sand prairie. At the close of the last Ice Age, the receding floodwaters left a vast amount of sand through this portion of the Illinois River valley. The winds sculpted the 100-foot dunes that became the wooded ridges the area is named for. This unique environment supports plant and animal species that are more typical of the Southwest than the Midwest, including prickly pear cactus.

Sand Ridge is also a great place to hike and camp if you want quiet and miles of forest trails to explore. As you enter on CR 2300 North, you'll find Pine Campground at the crossroads with Cactus Drive, situated within the shade of a beautiful grove of tall pines. Water spigots and vault toilets are conveniently located, and each site has a table and a ground grill. Over the holidays it may be close to full, but most other weekends you won't have more than a handful of neighbors.

Pitch your tent on a thick bed of soft pine needles at Pine Campground.

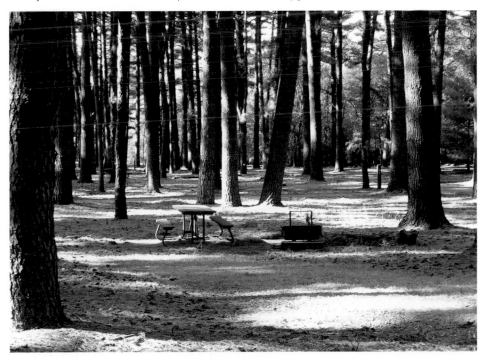

KEY INFORMATION

LOCATION: 25799 East CR 2300 North, Forest City, IL 61532

CONTACT: 309-597-2212, bit.ly/SandRidgeIL

OPERATED BY: IDNR

OPEN: Year-round (except firearm deer season, late November–early December)

SITES: Class C: 23 sites; Class C equestrian: 20 sites; Class D: 12 hike-in sites

EACH SITE HAS: Table, ground grill

WHEELCHAIR ACCESS: Restrooms and at least one accessible tent site

ASSIGNMENT: First come, first served; reservations available online

REGISTRATION: Register, then park staff will come by; register at office for hike-in sites

AMENITIES: Water spigot, vault toilets at Class C campsites only

PARKING: At campsite; nearest parking lot or roadside (hike-in sites)

FEE: Class C: $8/night; Class D: $6/night; $5 reservation fee

ELEVATION: 499'

RESTRICTIONS:

PETS: On leash only

QUIET HOURS: 10 p.m.–7 a.m.

FIRES: In fire rings only

ALCOHOL: Not permitted

VEHICLES: 2 per site

The 23 sites are laid out in three small loops, labeled A, B, and C, from east to west. A few sites are a bit small or too close to adjacent sites, but most are otherwise good choices. I prefer the sites on the outside and back of each loop because they tend to be larger and better shaded, as well as those in loop C because it's farther from the campground entrance. Site C5 is tucked away in its own bit of woods; B6 is my favorite—it's off the road and is the most spacious. You can reserve a site online, or simply pick an unreserved site on arrival, set up, and staff will come by for registration.

Sand Ridge also has 12 secluded hike-in campsites scattered throughout the forest; the closest is about 0.25 mile from the nearest parking. Each has a fire ring but no water or other facilities. Most are in wooded settings, out of sight of the trail, and have enough room for several tents. Before camping, you must register at the park office, open 8 a.m.–4 p.m. daily. If you arrive after office hours, camp at Pine Campground the first night and arrange for hike-in camping the next day. You can park at the lot closest to your site, or along the road, as long as you don't block a fire lane or trail, and all wheels are off the road. Pick up a trail map from the information kiosk at park headquarters. Nine of the hike-in sites can also be reserved online.

One attractive wooded hike-in site is BC 4, located on a small hill and off the trail. To get there, go 0.4 mile south from the crossroads of CR 2300 and Cactus Drive. Park off the road, and pick up the red trail on the west side of the road. After about 700 feet you come to the junction with the orange trail; turn right, and continue another 2,000 feet to the campsite, on the left, a total hike of about 0.5 mile.

Whether you want a little hiking or a lot, you'll find something suitable at Sand Ridge. The woods and interspersed meadows are beautiful and quiet. In the late spring or early summer, you may see the abundant prickly pear cactus in bloom, with their waxy yellow flowers. The fall offers the changing leaves, in all their colorful radiance. With about 44 miles of trail available, you can hike all day and rarely meet another person. The trail system

Sand Ridge State Forest

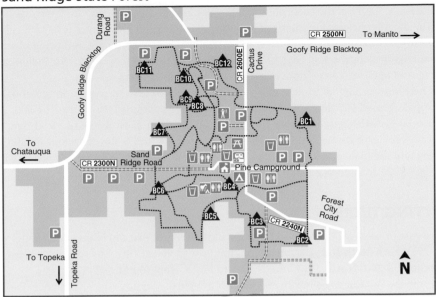

Sand Ridge State Forest: Pine Campground

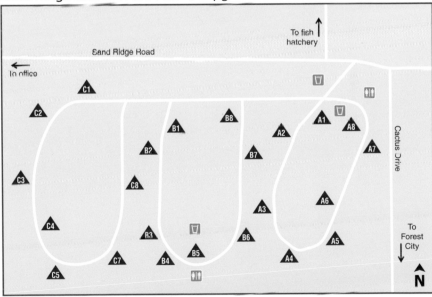

is composed of seven interconnecting loops, each blazed in a different color. The shortest loop is 1.25 miles long, and the longest is about 17 miles, with all sorts of possible routes between them. If that's not enough, there are also more than 120 miles of unmarked fire lanes that are not on the trail map—bring a compass or GPS if you want to hike these.

Otherwise, stick to the trails, and remember that they'll cross the wider fire lanes at various points. Note that equestrians may also share most of the trails within the trail system—the 2-mile green loop and the backcountry campsites are closed to horses.

The biggest challenge in hiking at Sand Ridge is the sand. The terrain is fairly level, but the sandy soil makes walking much more strenuous. Plan accordingly, and bring plenty of water. Hiking along the trail edge provides firmer footing in places. Watch for indentations in the sand made by horses' hooves, which can be ankle-twisters.

There's no fishing at Sand Ridge—water doesn't stay on the surface long enough to even make a mud puddle—but you can tour the state's largest fish hatchery. The Jake Wolf Memorial Fish Hatchery operates year-round and is open daily, 8:30 a.m.–3:30 p.m. The upper-level visitor center overlooks the operation below and features various exhibits on fishing and the pioneer life of the Illinois River valley. Tours are by appointment only; call 309-968-7531 to arrange a visit.

GETTING THERE

From east or west, take US 136 to CR 2800 East (12 miles east of Havana or 20 miles west of I-155). Turn north and go 6 miles straight, through Forest City. The road turns west and becomes CR 2300 North. Continue 2 miles to Pine Campground.

From the Peoria area, follow IL 29 south from Pekin to Manito Road. Turn right (west) and go 13.5 miles south into Manito. Turn right again onto CR 2500 North (Goofy Ridge Road). Drive 4.1 miles to Cactus Drive, then turn left (south) and go 2 miles to Pine Campground.

GPS COORDINATES: N40° 23.444'   W89° 51.991'

⛺ Siloam Springs State Park

Beauty ★★★ Privacy ★★★ Spaciousness ★★★ Quiet ★★★★ Security ★★★★ Cleanliness ★★★★★

Let your impatient younger anglers try out the Kid's Pond, where catches of 10–15 fish per half hour are common.

Rarely have I had to stop for deer more frequently in Illinois than I did driving through Siloam Springs State Park. With 3,323 acres, there's plenty of room for wildlife, and white-tailed deer and wild turkey are a common sight. The four main campgrounds at Siloam Springs also provide plenty of options for campers, who can spread out and choose the setting that best suits them.

As you enter the park, take the first right and pass the group campground to reach Hickory Hill Campground. To me, these 33 sites are not as attractive as those in the Pine Grove and Oak Ridge Campgrounds—but they're also not as busy. If you want fewer neighbors and don't mind driving to the showers, this is a good place. Here you'll find more singles and couples camping, and fewer families.

You can rent boats at the concession at Siloam Springs.

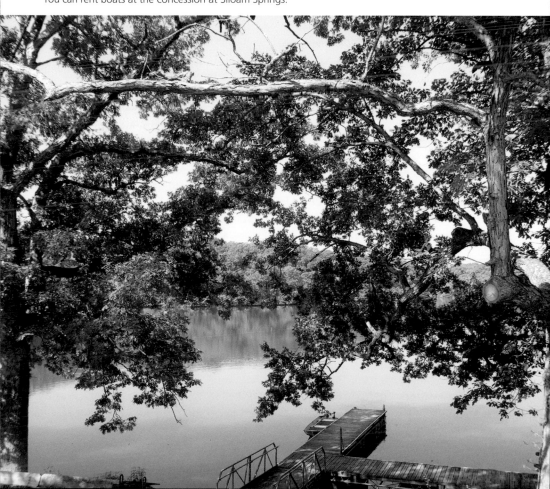

KEY INFORMATION

LOCATION: 938 East 3003rd Lane, Clayton, IL 62324

CONTACT: 217-894-6205, bit.ly/SiloamSpringsIL

OPERATED BY: IDNR

OPEN: Year-round

SITES: Class A: 91 electric sites; Class B: 30 nonelectric sites; 4 backpacking sites; 28 equestrian-only sites

EACH SITE HAS: Picnic table, ground grill; electricity at Class A only

WHEELCHAIR ACCESS: Restrooms and at least one accessible tent site

ASSIGNMENT: First come, first served; reservations available online (Pine Grove and Oak Ridge only)

REGISTRATION: Select site, then register with the campground host or at the office

AMENITIES: Water spigots, vault toilets, shower house

PARKING: At site; in lot (walk-in sites); at park office (backpacking sites)

FEE: Class A: $20/night, $30/night holidays; Class B: $10/night; backpacking: $8/night; $5 reservation fee

ELEVATION: 684'

RESTRICTIONS:

PETS: On leash only

QUIET HOURS: 10 p.m.–7 a.m.

FIRES: In fire rings only

ALCOHOL: Permitted

VEHICLES: 2 per site

OTHER: 14-day limit; 1 RV and 1 tent, or 2 tents per site; 4 adults or 1 family per site

Most of these sites are electric, and, peculiar to Siloam Springs, tents at electric sites must be pitched on the square gravel tent pads, not on the grass. This does provide a nice, flat, raised surface, but I prefer natural earth beneath my tent. Fortunately, Hickory Hill features 11 nonelectric grass tent sites on the south side of this elongated loop, set off in three sections up against the woods. You can't park at each site, but the farthest is only about 50 feet away. Circle the loop counterclockwise, and you'll come first to my favorite set of sites, 9B, 10B, and 11B. There's plenty of space, and you're as far from other campers as you can be here. Site 11B is the most popular, well shaded by two massive oak trees. It's also right by the 0.25-mile Raccoon Trail, which leads down to a floating dock on the lake, where you can fish or simply sit and watch the sun rise. Don't pitch your tent right by the trailhead, though, unless you like having other campers trudge through your campsite.

If any of these first three sites is taken, move down to the next set (6B–8B) or the third (1B–5B). On an average nonholiday weekend you have a good chance of getting one of these sections to yourself.

Another alternative for tent campers is the group campground, which you pass on the way to Hickory Hill. When the sites are not reserved or occupied by a group, individuals can pick one of the dozen or so unnumbered nonelectric sites in this grassy area. These aren't as well shaded, but if you want more privacy this is a good choice. The weekend I camped at Hickory Hill, there was one lone camper in the group area. Note that Hickory Hill and the group campground close from November 1–late May.

Farther into the park, you'll find the entrance to Pine Grove and Oak Ridge Campgrounds, along the same road. These are busier, with more RVs, but they're also more scenic and closer to the showers. As you drive in, Pine Grove is particularly striking, with well-laid-out sites set beneath tall, stately pines. Of the 76 sites in these two areas, 17 are designated tent-only, and 10 of these are electric, scattered among the RV sites. In the first loop they are 9, 10, 11, 14, 16, 17, and 24; in the second, 41 and 56; and in the third, 71. If you want electricity, the most attractive and spacious of these are 9, 10, and 11. However, to me the nicest for tent camping are the nonelectric sites 61–64, all by themselves down the road in Oak Ridge. The other nonelectric sites in Oak Ridge are 77, 80, and 81. Each has a table, fire ring, and lantern pole.

Fishing is a prime draw at Siloam Springs, particularly at the start of the trout seasons, the first Saturday in April, and the third Saturday in October. You can bank or boat fish, or cast a line from one of the six floating docks around the 58-acre lake. The Boathouse concession sells bait, tackle, ice, firewood, snacks, and a few sandwich and breakfast items. You can also rent paddleboats, pontoon boats, canoes, kayaks, and rowboats with trolling motors there. They're open April–Labor Day, 6 a.m.–6 p.m., Tuesday–Thursday and Sunday, and until 9 p.m. Friday and Saturday (then shorter hours through October). Phone 217-894-6263 for more information.

If you have impatient younger anglers, let them test the waters at the Kid's Pond, right by the park entrance. They can bank fish almost all the way around the pond, and catches of 10–15 redear and bluegill per half hour are common.

You can explore Siloam Springs' forested ridges via about 12 miles of hiking trails. The most challenging is the 4-mile Red Oak Backpack Trail, with steep slopes and several creek crossings. If you really want to get away, there are four primitive campsites with fire pits, tables, and a pit toilet, about midway along the loop. To camp there, register first and leave your vehicle at the park office, then take Deer Run Trail to the Red Oak trailhead, adding another mile to the hike. Avoid this trail when it's wet, though—it can get very muddy.

Siloam Springs State Park

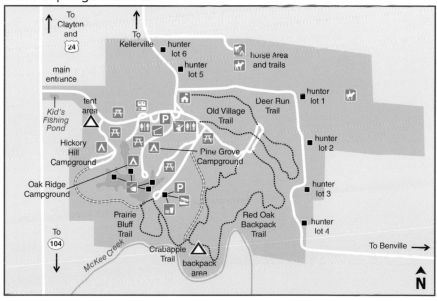

Siloam Springs State Park: Hickory Hill Campground

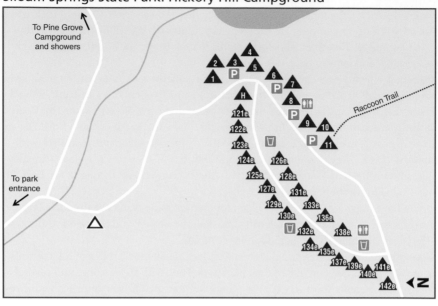

Siloam Springs State Park: Pine Grove and Oak Ridge Campgrounds

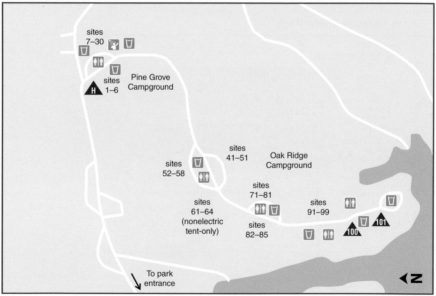

GETTING THERE

From Mount Sterling, take US 24 west about 10 miles to CR 2950 East, just before Clayton. Turn left, go 7 miles south to the three-way stop at Kellerville. Turn left onto CR 1200 North and drive 1.1 miles, then make a left on CR 2873 South and travel 2.4 miles south to the park entrance, on the left.

From Springfield, take I-72 west to Exit 35 (Griggsville). Head 11 miles north on IL 107 to IL 104, then take a left. Drive 12 miles to CR 2873 East, then hang a right and travel 5.8 miles to the park entrance, on the right.

GPS COORDINATES: N39° 53.756'   W90° 57.284'

Pitch your tent beneath the tall pines at Pine Grove Campground.

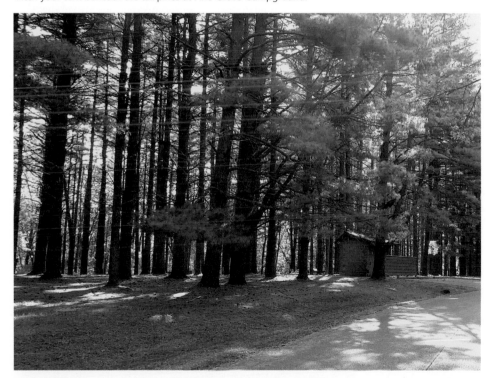

25

Spring Lake State Fish and Wildlife Area

Beauty ★★★ Privacy ★★★ Spaciousness ★★★ Quiet ★★★★ Security ★★★★ Cleanliness ★★★★★

Camp beneath towering pines, with a bed of soft pine needles under your tent.

The Illinois River valley has been attracting visitors for more than 10,000 years, when the first American Indians settled there to take advantage of the abundant wildlife, water, and fertile soil. Today a number of parks and wildlife refuges continue to draw hunters, anglers, birders, and campers to the area. One of the prettiest places to camp is beneath the oak or pine trees at Spring Lake State Fish and Wildlife Area. The park offers two quite different camping areas, separated from each other by several miles, and ample opportunities for wildlife viewing and fishing.

The narrow, shallow lake that makes up two-thirds of Spring Lake's 2,032 acres is an abandoned channel of the Illinois River and runs parallel to the river for about 8 miles on its eastern side. These are the river's bottomlands, but the lake is bordered on the east by a large sandstone bluff, and the park's campgrounds, office, and hiking trails are on that side, about 80 feet above the lake level. The lake is divided into northern and southern sections by an east–west causeway.

The walk-in camping area is at the southern end of the lake, near the office. Register and park there, then cross the road to one of the six sites—three close to the road, and three up on the grass-covered hill. The sites are spread out, though they don't have much shade or brush between them. I suggest walking the extra distance to the sites farthest out, as the others are within sight of the park maintenance building—kind of like camping near a garage. Each site has a picnic table and a fire ring; there are vault toilets nearby, and there's

Pine Campground is my favorite place to camp at Spring Lake.

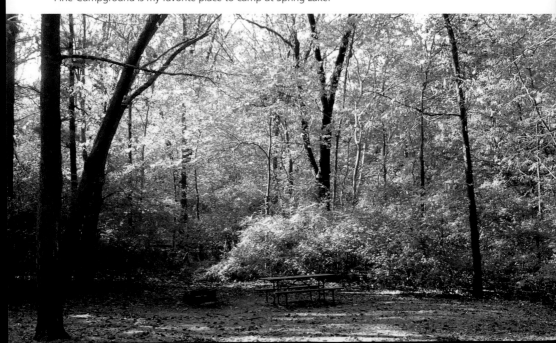

KEY INFORMATION

LOCATION: 7982 South Park Road, Manito, IL 61546

CONTACT: 309-968-7135, bit.ly/SpringLakeIL

OPERATED BY: IDNR

OPEN: Year-round

SITES: Class C: 60 vehicle-accessible sites; Class D: 6 walk-in tent sites

EACH SITE HAS: Picnic table, fire ring

WHEELCHAIR ACCESS: Not designated

ASSIGNMENT: First come, first served

REGISTRATION: Set up and park staff will come by (Class C); register at the office (Class D)

AMENITIES: Water spigots, vault toilets

PARKING: At site (Class C); in lot (Class D)

FEE: Class C: $8/night; Class D: $6/night

ELEVATION: 505'

RESTRICTIONS:

PETS: On leash only

QUIET HOURS: 10 p.m.–7 a.m.

FIRES: In fire rings only

ALCOHOL: Not permitted

VEHICLES: 2 per site

OTHER: 14-day limit; 1 RV or 2 tents per site; 4 adults or 1 family per site

a water spigot by the road. This area also doubles as the group campground, used by youth groups about 10 weekends a year. Though not required to do so, most groups notify the office in advance, so you can ask if any are scheduled before deciding to camp there.

As a tent camper, my first inclination is to go for the walk-in sites—I assume they'll be more secluded, more attractive, and less used. At Spring Lake, however, I prefer the vehicular access sites at the northern end of the lake. They're much prettier, well shaded, and usually not busy. From the office, head 3.25 miles north to the causeway, cross the lake, and continue 1.75 miles on Spring Lake Road to the northern campground entrance, on the left. One quarter-mile in you'll come to an intersection and have to make a choice: Oak Campground on the right, or Pine Campground on the left? Both are aptly named. The 38 sites along the Oak loop sit beneath spreading oaks, with a few pines thrown in and some trees and brush separating the sites from one another. Head toward the back of the loop, where the sites are roomier—I like 18 and 20.

Pine is the smaller of the two loops, with 22 sites, and is definitely my favorite place to camp at Spring Lake. It's a rare treat to camp beneath towering pines in Illinois—I love the scent and the bed of soft pine needles under the tent. Some sites on the northern outside of the loop are a bit hilly, but the rest are excellent. Site 51, at the far end, probably offers the most space and distance from neighboring sites. Site 60, on the left near the entrance, is also larger, and 57 and 58, while smaller, are tucked away from view.

All sites have a table and a fire ring, and there are water spigots and vault toilets nearby. Just pitch your tent, and park staff will come by to register you later. You'll never have trouble finding a spot here—the campground never completely fills up, even on holiday weekends. On most fair-weather nonholiday weekends, about one-third of the 60 sites will be occupied, whether by tents or by smaller RVs.

Fishing is a prime attraction at Spring Lake, particularly in the spring, before the growth of aquatic vegetation makes it more challenging. The north lake is better suited to boat fishing, and largemouth bass and muskie are among the targets. The south lake has plenty of well-mown spots for bank fishing, and these can be accessed from the six parking areas along the 2-mile stretch of road from the causeway south. Besides the typical bass, bluegill, crappie, and channel catfish, south lake's cool spring-fed waters support a healthy population of northern pike. There's a nice picnic area at the southern end of the lake and a fish-cleaning station at the boat ramp along the causeway.

For an educational adventure, take a trip back in time at the Dickson Mounds Museum, about 30 miles to the southwest, across the Illinois River near Lewiston. Interactive exhibits, multimedia presentations, and the excavated remains of American Indian buildings highlight the prehistory of the Illinois River valley. Be sure to go up on the roof for a panoramic view of the area. The museum is free and open daily. Check bit.ly/DicksonMoundsIL for more details.

Spring Lake State Fish and Wildlife Area: North Campgrounds

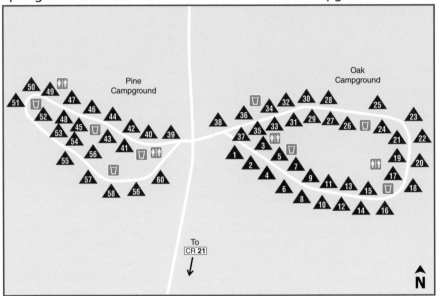

GETTING THERE

From Pekin, take IL 29 south about 1 mile to Manito Road. Turn right (west) and go 10.3 miles to Spring Lake Road. Turn right again and travel 3.1 miles west to the north campground entrance, on the right. To get to the office, continue west on Spring Lake Road 1.75 miles across the lake, turn left, and go 3.25 miles south.

GPS COORDINATES: N40° 27.900'   W89° 50.549' **(NORTH CAMPGROUND ENTRANCE)**

26

⚠ Walnut Point State Park

Beauty ★★★★ Privacy ★★★★ Spaciousness ★★★★ Quiet ★★★★ Security ★★★★ Cleanliness ★★★★

The campgrounds at Walnut Point provide easy access for fishing or boating and afford a scenic view right from your campsite.

Like the fingers of an outstretched hand, the little peninsulas on which the campgrounds at Walnut Point State Park are situated jut out into the beautiful 60-acre lake, providing easy access for fishing or boating, and affording a scenic view right from your campsite. In some cases you can row up to your site or fish at a dock just a few steps from your tent. This small park boasts 60 sites, but they are spread out in separate loops, so they don't have the typical "sardines-in-a-can" campground feel. The tent-only campsites are walk-ins—close enough to parking to be convenient but far enough that they're not as popular as the pull-in sites. And tent campers can use the showers—a nice perk.

Enter Walnut Point from the north, turn left, and follow the loop around the lake to the back of the park, where the campgrounds are. Over the dam and past the concession, you'll

Looking out over the lake at Walnut Point

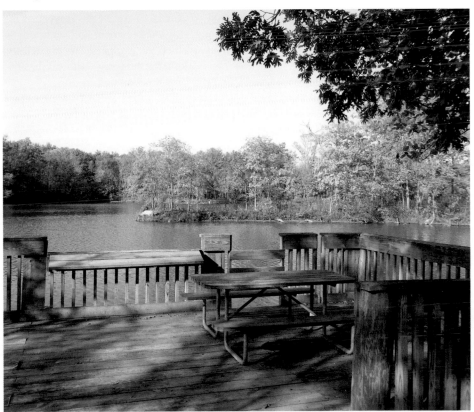

KEY INFORMATION

LOCATION: 2331 East CR 370 North, Oakland, IL 61943

CONTACT: 217-346-3336, bit.ly/WalnutPointIL

OPERATED BY: IDNR

OPEN: Year-round

SITES: Class A: 34 electric sites; Class B: 6 sites; Class C: 20 walk-in sites

EACH SITE HAS: Picnic tables, fire ring and grate

WHEELCHAIR ACCESS: Restrooms and at least one accessible tent site

ASSIGNMENT: First come, first served; reservations available online for Class A and C

REGISTRATION: Register with the campground host or set up and park staff will come by

AMENITIES: Water spigots, vault toilets, shower house (closed November 1–May 1)

PARKING: At site (Class A & B); at lot (Class C)

FEE: Class A: $20/night, $30/night on holidays; Class B: $13/night; Class C: $8/night; $5 reservation fee

ELEVATION: 657'

RESTRICTIONS:

PETS: On leash only

QUIET HOURS: 10 p.m.–7 a.m.

FIRES: In fire rings only

ALCOHOL: Not permitted at Class C sites

VEHICLES: 2 per site

OTHER: 14-day limit; 1 RV and 1 tent, or 2 tents per site; 4 adults or 1 family per site; no swimming

see the entrance to Fox Squirrel Campground. Pull-in sites 1–14 are on this drive; parking for the walk-in tent sites is just opposite site 10, along with a water spigot and vault toilets.

Past Fox Squirrel is the modern shower house, which all campers can use (closed November 1–May 1). Farther on the right you'll see parking for the Gray Tent walk-in sites, and beyond that, at the end of the road, you'll find the Gray Squirrel pull-in sites.

The best choices for tent camping are the 20 walk-in sites in the Fox Tent and Gray Tent areas. All have two picnic tables, a wood-chipped tent pad, a ground grill or fire ring, and a lantern post. Holidays may find these areas fairly full, but less than half will be occupied on most other good camping weekends.

Walk 250 feet from the Fox Tent parking lot to the end of the peninsula, where you'll see lots of space surrounding sites 7 and 8, the two most scenic sites in this area. Here you'll find plenty of shade, an unobstructed view of the lake, and a dock right off site 7. Site 5 is a bit farther back from the trail than the others. Site 1 is wheelchair accessible, and just behind site 2 is an accessible dock and fishing platform.

I like the sites in Gray Tent best. Site 20, a 350-foot walk to the end of the peninsula, boasts a great view and plenty of room to spread out. If you want something a bit closer, sites 11 and 13 are less than 100 feet from parking, off a dogleg to the right of the trail. These feel more secluded. Site 13 also has a dock and is the single most popular of all the walk-ins. If your group needs two adjacent sites, check out the combination of sites 16 and 18, which are close to one another but separate from the others.

If you want electricity, the best Class A sites are at the back of the Gray Squirrel loop—sites 15, 17, and 19 on the outside of the loop offer ample space for a tent, shade, and proximity to the lake; there's a dock just behind site 15. The sites in Fox Squirrel loop are not as spacious; site 5 is probably the best choice there for space and shade, though it's close to the restroom.

Walnut Point State Park

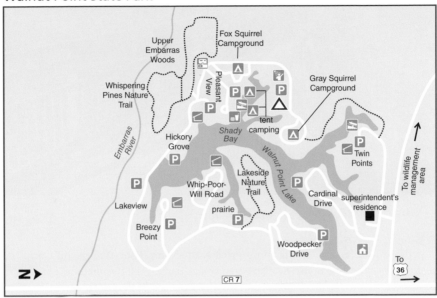

Walnut Point State Park: Fox Squirrel and Gray Squirrel Campgrounds

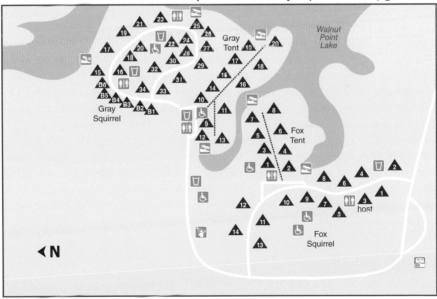

If you want a pull-in site but don't need electricity, sites B1–B6 at the entrance to the Gray Squirrel loop aren't bad. B1, B2, and B3 have space for a pop-up trailer to back in and feature a cleared, wood-chipped pad for a tent.

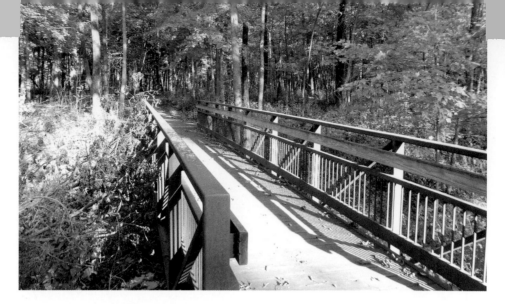
The paved 0.5-mile Woodpecker Trail is wheelchair accessible.

For those wanting something more private, the Whip-Poor-Will group camp on the opposite side of the lake is also available to any size party. Facilities include a vault toilet, a shelter, two docks, and a pier. There is no water or showers, but campers can use both at the other campgrounds. The cost is $2/person/night ($20 minimum) if kids are in your party or $4/person/night ($40 minimum) for an all-adult group.

All the Class A and Class C sites at Walnut Point can be reserved online through reserveamerica.com for an additional $5, which is probably a good idea on weekends. Otherwise, register with the campground host (if available) on arrival, or pick an unreserved site and set up, and park staff will come by.

For a woodland hike with a destination, try the aptly named Whispering Pines Trail. Hike the loop counterclockwise, and watch for signs for the Observatory Trail. This 2.55-mile trek leads you past a three-story domed concrete bunker: an observatory built by the University of Illinois in the late 1960s. While it no longer functions and you can't go in, it is interesting and unusual to see.

Williams Cafe at Shady Bay serves as a popular gathering point and is open daily except for Monday from April 1 through the end of October. There you can purchase firewood, ice, and bait, and rent rowboats and paddleboats. The restaurant offers plenty of snack and meal choices, including daily specials and homemade desserts. You can eat there, indoors or out, or get takeout. Call 217-346-2005 for more information or check their Facebook page: bit.ly/FB-WilliamsCafe.

GETTING THERE

From I-57 at Tuscola, take Exit 212. Follow US 36 East 13 miles. Turn right onto CR 2360 East at the Walnut Point sign and drive 6 miles south. Turn right onto CR 400 North. Drive 0.25 mile to the park entrance, on the left.

GPS COORDINATES: N39° 42.305'   W88° 01.830'

27

Weldon Springs State Park

Beauty ★★★★★ Privacy ★★★★ Spaciousness ★★★ Quiet ★★★★ Security ★★★★★ Cleanliness ★★★★★

Take time to linger at the impressive Veterans Point along the scenic 2-mile lakeside trail.

I still remember my first visits to Weldon Springs as a kid—picnicking by the lake, fishing with my family, and my brother catching a snapping turtle that he wanted to bring home.

This gem of the Illinois State Parks System is still a very family-friendly place. Kids and adults will enjoy the scenic 29-acre lake, with plenty of bluegill and crappie to catch. The park's 550 acres feature well-maintained, easy hiking trails, excellent playgrounds, picnic shelters, sand volleyball courts, and even a little nature museum and vintage schoolhouse.

Two miles of road circle the lake and provide access to most of the park. The second right after you enter leads to the campground, where you'll find the host's trailer, along with an information board with park maps. Register with the host, if available; otherwise, pick an unreserved site, set up, and register at the self-registration post there.

The campground is clean and comfortable, with 75 Class A sites with electricity and limited shade. The shower house is open to all campers May–October (weather permitting). If you'd like the convenience of parking where you camp but don't need electricity, there are 4 Class B sites (79–82) on the western edge of the campground loop.

Veterans Point along the lake trail honors more than 1,400 veterans.

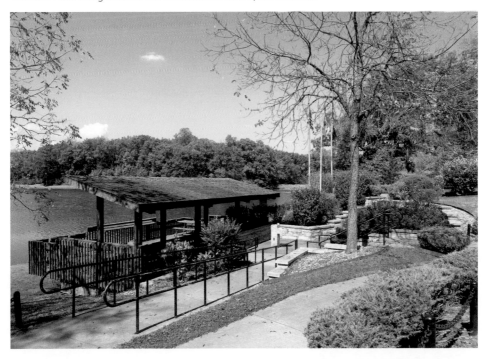

KEY INFORMATION

LOCATION: 4734 Weldon Springs Road, Clinton IL 61727

CONTACT: 217-935-2644, bit.ly/WeldonSpringsIL

OPERATED BY: IDNR

OPEN: Year-round

SITES: Class A: 75 sites; Class B: 4 sites; Class C: 15 walk-in/backpack sites

EACH SITE HAS: Picnic table, ground grill; electricity at Class A only

WHEELCHAIR ACCESS: Restrooms and at least one accessible tent site

ASSIGNMENT: First come, first served; reservations available online

REGISTRATION: Register with camp host

AMENITIES: Water spigots, vault toilets; shower house (open May–October)

PARKING: At site; in lot (walk-in sites)

FEE: Class A: $20/night, $30/night holidays; Class B: $10/night; Class C: $8/night

ELEVATION: 611'

RESTRICTIONS:

PETS: On leash only

FIRES: In fire rings only

ALCOHOL: Prohibited in tent/backpack sites and group camp

VEHICLES: 2 per site

OTHER: 14-day limit; 1 RV and 1 tent, or 2 tents per site; 4 adults or 1 family per site

---

Park across from the host's trailer to access the nine walk-in tent sites. These are close to one another but surrounded by enough woods and brush to give some sense of privacy. Each has a picnic table and fire ring. Sites 1, 2, and 6 are close to the road, and 4 is smaller. Site 3 is fairly spacious. Site 10 is at the back, but right on the trail to the lake. My favorites here are 8 and 9.

The real beauties for tent campers wanting more privacy are the six little-used "backpacking" sites along the Salt Creek Backpack Trail. However, don't think "backpacking" means lugging your gear for miles. The first four sites are located within 150 feet of the parking area.

After registering, proceed in either direction around the park loop to Lookout Point Road. Go to the picnic area and park in the first spots past the sign. The Salt Creek Backpack Trail begins to the left and downhill. Sites 1–4 are ahead, each with a table and fire ring. Site 1 is my favorite—it's the most spacious and the farthest off the trail. Sites 2 and 3 are smaller, across the trail from each other. The terrain slopes a bit on site 4, making it less ideal for tents.

Backpack campers can use the toilets and water spigot at the picnic area, as well as the campground's shower facilities. And the Lookout Point picnic area is well named; it commands an impressive view eastward over the Salt Creek valley. It's worth the effort to wake up early, climb the hill to the pavilion, and watch the sunrise.

If you want more seclusion and don't mind hiking a bit, head for the two backpack sites down by Salt Creek. The trail is wide and an easy 1-mile hike. A park naturalist told me that she and her kids used to throw all their camping gear in a wagon and simply pull it behind—the trail is that smooth. However, the backpack trail is intersected at several points by cross-country skiing trails, so it's easy to get lost.

From the first four sites, head downhill. Past the bottom of the hill, turn left at the first intersection. Facing the bench there, take the trail to the right. At the next two forks, take the right again. You'll eventually see a sign with a backpacker symbol. Take the left fork as indicated, and the first site will be directly ahead. The second is another 100 yards farther. Both are beautiful, spacious, grassy sites with a table and fire ring, right on the banks of the Salt Creek. These sites can flood in the spring—call first to be sure they're available.

Though it is usually unnecessary for the tent-only sites except for holidays, any site at Weldon Springs can be reserved online. Note that "holiday" also includes the last full weekend of September, during Clinton's annual Apple 'n Pork Festival.

One of my favorite short hikes in central Illinois is the scenic 2-mile trail that circles the lake. It's easy and varied enough for kids, and there are lots of fishing platforms and several restrooms along the way. Depending on the time of year, you're likely to see geese, turtles, and blue heron. Take time to linger at the impressive Veterans Point Memorial on the east side. The covered overlook, bronze statue, and granite stones honoring more than 1,400 veterans were built entirely from private donations.

If you're there on a weekend, young naturalists will also love a visit to the Union School Interpretive Center. The two buildings include a restored one-room school built in 1865 and a small but packed nature museum with "please touch" exhibits. The center is staffed by volunteers, so hours may vary, but most recently it was open from Memorial Day through Labor Day on Saturday and Sunday, noon–3 p.m.

There is one family favorite that the park doesn't have: swimming. However, you can drive the 15 miles or so to Clinton Lake State Recreation Area, where for $2 you can swim all day on a beautiful sandy beach, with shower house and concession.

Begin the 2-mile trail that circles the lake here.

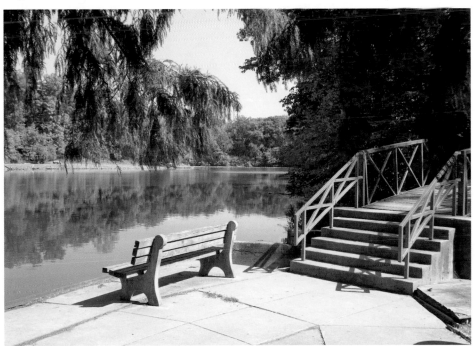

Weldon Springs State Park

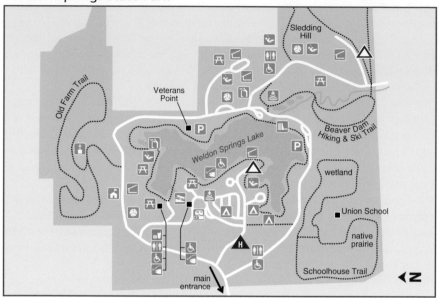

Weldon Springs State Park Campground

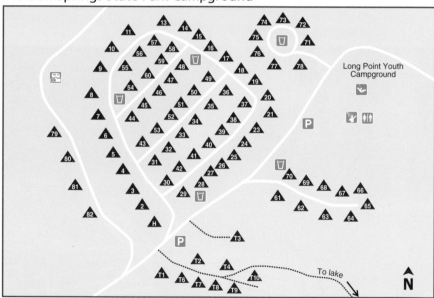

Weldon Springs State Park: Lookout Point Backpack Campsites

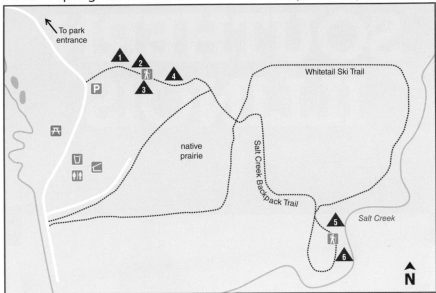

GETTING THERE

From Decatur, take US 51 north about 15 miles to Clinton. Turn right onto Business 51 at the first stop light, then take the very next right onto Revere Rd. Go 1 mile to CR 18, turn right, and continue 1.3 miles to the park entrance on the left.

GPS COORDINATES: N40° 07.314'   W88° 55.915'

SOUTHERN ILLINOIS

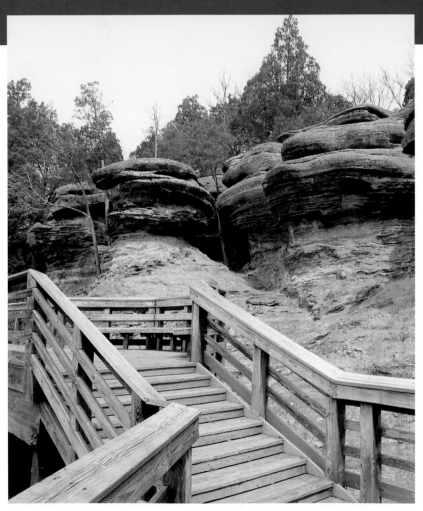

The Observation Trail winds among fantastic rock formations at Garden of the Gods (see page 134).

28

⚠ Beall Woods State Park

Beauty ★★ Privacy ★★★ Spaciousness ★★★ Quiet ★★★ Security ★★★★ Cleanliness ★★★★★

In this Midwestern equivalent of California's redwood forest, some 300 trees grow to more than 120 feet tall.

You can visit Dickson Mounds, Cahokia Mounds, Millstone Bluff, and other places in Illinois to view artifacts of the American Indians who lived here long before Europeans came. At Beall (pronounced "bell") Woods State Park, however, you can see what the woodlands themselves looked like in those pre-pioneer days. Within the 635 acres of this park on the banks of the Wabash River are 329 acres of old-growth woods—virtually untouched by man—the largest remnant of the original deciduous forests that once covered perhaps 40% of the state. In this Midwestern equivalent of California's redwood forest, some 300 trees grow to more than 120 feet tall.

For the sake of the centuries-old trees, however, you cannot camp in the woods. The campground is a simple half loop of 16 sites, set along the edge of a flat, open field near the park's entrance. A line of trees stands behind the sites to the west, but there isn't a lot of shade where you camp. I wouldn't call it scenic, but there's plenty of space, it's clean, and it's not real busy outside of holidays. On an average weekend perhaps four or five sites will be occupied. There's room for RVs to park, but since there's no electricity or showers, you probably won't see more than the occasional pop-up camper.

Check out the educational exhibits in the excellent visitor center.

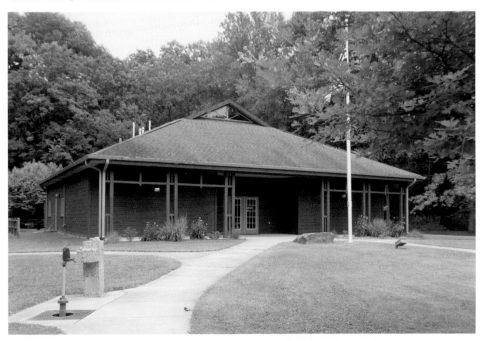

KEY INFORMATION

LOCATION: 9285 Beall Woods Ave., Mount Carmel, IL 62863

CONTACT: 618-298-2442, bit.ly/BeallWoodsIL

OPERATED BY: IDNR

OPEN: Year-round

SITES: Class C: 16

EACH SITE HAS: Picnic table, ground grill

WHEELCHAIR ACCESS: Restrooms and at least one accessible tent site

ASSIGNMENT: First come, first served

REGISTRATION: Set up first, then park staff will come by

AMENITIES: Water spigots, vault toilets

PARKING: At site

FEE: $8/night

ELEVATION: 407'

RESTRICTIONS:

PETS: On leash only

QUIET HOURS: 10 p.m.–7 a.m.

FIRES: In fire rings only

ALCOHOL: Not permitted

VEHICLES: 2 per site

OTHER: 14-day limit; 1 RV and 1 tent, or 2 tents per site; 4 adults or 1 family per site

As you enter the park, the campground is on the left. The campground road is one-way, from north to south, so head past the southern end to enter from the north. I prefer the sites on the right, outside the loop; sites 6, 8, and 9, in the middle, are even more spread out. Site 14, toward the end, is nicely shaded. Each site has one or two tables; vault toilets and a water spigot are centrally located, across from site 9. Registration is simple—just set up, and park staff will come by later.

You come to Beall Woods to see the trees, of course. Start your exploration at the excellent visitor center, where you can pick up a trail map and see the interactive exhibits on the history and ecology of the area. This is a kid-friendly place—many school groups come here each year for environmental education programs. Additionally, the site interpreter leads a variety of free nature hikes and activities, some especially for kids and requiring advance registration. Check the website for scheduled activities. The visitor center is open Sunday and Monday noon–4 p.m. and 8 a.m.–4 p.m. the rest of the week.

Five loop trails, totaling 6.25 miles, wander through the woods, along Coffee and Sugar Creeks, and by the wide Wabash River. This portion of Beall Woods is an Illinois nature preserve and a federally designated national landmark, so pets, bicycles, and horses are not allowed, and hikers should stay on the established trails to protect the natural resources (and avoid the large patches of poison ivy). The trails are easy to hike and well marked—the only hazard is that you could walk into a ravine as you gawk at the trees overhead. Of the 64 species of trees in the park, 2—sugarberry (125 feet) and shellbark hickory (135 feet)—have their state champions at Beall Woods. Hundreds of others, while not the tallest of their species, reach awe-inspiring height and girth. (For a complete list of Illinois's largest trees by species, and the GPS locations for some, check bit.ly/BigTreesIL.)

Two trails begin just behind the visitor center. The 1-mile Tuliptree Trail is the easiest, circling through upland woods and along a small bluff over Coffee Creek. White Oak Trail is 1.25 miles long—moderately easy, with a couple flights of steps—and is one of the best for viewing the large trees. From the southern tip of White Oak you can cross a bridge over Coffee Creek to access the 1.75-mile Ridgway Trail, which passes through a reforested field along the Wabash River. The 0.5-mile Sweet Gum and 1.75-mile Schenck Trails are north of Coffee Creek. You can reach them from a separate parking lot north of the main entrance: Exit the park, turn right, then immediately make another right onto CR 800 East; proceed 1.3 miles north to the lot on the right as the road curves left. Note that the Ridgway, Sweet Gum, and Schenck Trails are closed when flooded.

Beall Woods also has a 15-acre lake where you can fish for bluegill, largemouth bass, and catfish and is among 43 in the state stocked with trout each spring and fall. The park occasionally hosts scout camping events and often welcomes school groups for day visits. These are always scheduled in advance, so if you want to camp (or just hike) in peace, I recommend calling first to find out if any large groups are on the calendar.

Beall Woods State Park Campground

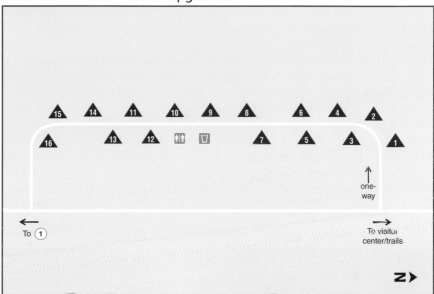

GETTING THERE

From I-64 at Exit 130, take IL 1 north 12 miles to Keensburg. Turn right on First Street (CR 16), then go 1 block to Market Street (CR 3) and turn left. Follow the road as it curves left and becomes CR 900 North; it's 2 miles to Beall Woods. From US 50 at IL 1 in Lawrenceville, take IL 1 south 33 miles to Keensburg. Turn left on First Street and proceed as above.

GPS COORDINATES: N38° 20.872'   W87° 50.091'

29

⚑ Bell Smith Springs Recreation Area:
RED BUD CAMPGROUND

Beauty ★★★★★ Privacy ★★★ Spaciousness ★★★ Quiet ★★★★★ Security ★★★★ Cleanliness ★★★★

This quiet little campground is a perfect base camp for exploring the superlative sites in the central Shawnee Forest.

Red Bud is a small, quiet, primitive campground in Bell Smith Springs Recreation Area, off a gravel road in the Shawnee National Forest. It's a great place for a relaxed getaway—but an even better base camp for exploring all the nearby superlative sites in the central Shawnee. Clustered within a few miles of this campground you'll find Illinois's highest waterfall, tallest natural arch, and largest sandstone cave, all within what some consider the most beautiful part of the Shawnee.

At you turn off McCormick Road toward Bell Smith Springs, you'll see a gated drive on the right. That's Teal Pond, formerly a campground but no longer maintained as such by the U.S. Forest Service. You can still fish there, but you'll have to hike the short distance past the gate to the three-acre pond.

Two miles farther down the road you'll come to the campground entrance, on the right. Red Bud Campground consists of a single loop with 21 well-shaded sites, each with a table, a fire ring, and a lantern post. Every site is large enough for a tent or two—I prefer sites 3 and 17 for space and shade. Though the sites aren't isolated from one another, the campground is usually not too busy. When I was there on a beautiful Saturday in June, only two

The creeks and rocks of Bell Smith Springs invite exploration. *photo by Oleksandr Koretskyi/Shutterstock*

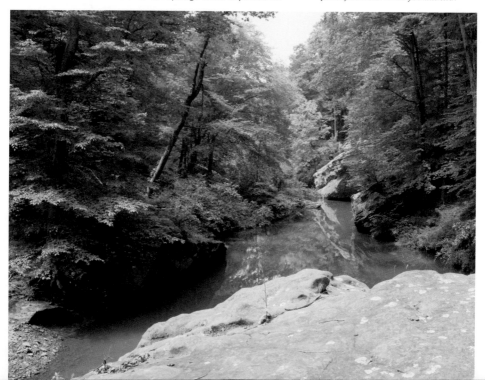

KEY INFORMATION

LOCATION: Bell Smith Springs Road, Ozark, IL 62972

CONTACT: Hidden Springs Ranger District, 618-658-2111, bit.ly/RedBudIL

OPERATED BY: U.S. Forest Service

OPEN: March 15–December 15

SITES: 21

EACH SITE HAS: Picnic table, fire ring, and lantern pole

WHEELCHAIR ACCESS: Not designated

ASSIGNMENT: First come, first served

REGISTRATION: Register at the self-registration post at the entrance

AMENITIES: Water spigot, vault toilets

PARKING: At site

FEE: $10/night

ELEVATION: 627'

RESTRICTIONS:

PETS: On leash only

QUIET HOURS: 10 p.m.–6 a.m.

FIRES: In fire rings only

ALCOHOL: Permitted

VEHICLES: 2 per site

OTHER: 14-day limit; 8 campers per site

---

sites were occupied. Take your pick of spots, set up camp, and pay at the self-registration post at the campground entrance.

Drive down the road just a short distance, and you'll come to the main trailhead parking for Bell Smith Springs, one of the most scenic areas in the entire Shawnee Forest. Here four creeks come together in a landscape of canyons, pools, boulders, and shelter caves. This area can be busy, at least on weekends, so plan to hike midweek if possible, or first thing in the morning. Three interconnecting loop trails begin here, and the fourth can be accessed from one of the others. Each is marked with color-coded diamonds, totaling about 8 miles of moderately rugged hiking. Particularly in the spring, you will ford creeks on slippery sandstone, so wear appropriate shoes. You'll find a trail map on the board at the parking area, but it's helpful to have a printed copy too—you can find one online at bit.ly /BellSmithSpringsMapIL.

Natural Bridge Trail, blazed in yellow, is a 1.5-mile loop that will take you above and below an impressive sandstone arch, 30 feet high and 125 feet long, the highest in the Shawnee Forest. You can climb to the top via the iron rungs anchored to the vertical face (installed back in the 1930s—be careful, one rung is loose!), or take the more circuitous and somewhat safer trail. The blue-blazed 3.2-mile Sentry Bluff loop leads along the cliff edge and down into the canyon to Boulder Falls. Parts of this trail toward the east end of the canyon are rugged and steep, so be prepared for a workout. It runs with Natural Bridge Trail at first, and the two can be combined. White diamonds mark the 1.4-mile General Trail, which leads past the Devil's Backbone ridge, by clear spring-fed pools—where some are inclined to take a dip on a hot summer day—and eventually to the spring itself. The 2-mile Mill Branch loop follows the creek canyon of the same name. It's blazed in orange and can be picked up from the end of the white trail or from the Hunting Branch Picnic Area (the first road right before the campground).

Illinois's highest waterfall, Burden Falls, is just 4 miles from the campground, in the Burden Falls Wilderness. Head back up to McCormick Road, turn left, drive 1.5 miles, turn right, and go 0.5 mile to the Burden Falls parking area. There's a smaller set of falls visible from the road, but the 100-foot falls are just a short hike from there. The water flow is very impressive in the spring. A 3.5-mile loop trail begins at the top of the falls, though you may want to get a topographic map before exploring it.

From the highest waterfall, you can head to the country's largest sandstone cave, Sand Cave. Turn left onto McCormick Road and drive 1.9 miles to Cedar Grove Road. Turn right, go 2.4 miles, and turn left just past Cedar Grove Church. Travel 0.2 mile to where you can park by the U.S. Forest Service sign. From there a 1-mile well-defined trail leads to the cave, which is about 100 feet long and 30 feet high.

And not far from Bell Smith Springs is the beautiful and rugged Jackson Hollow, the rock climber's mecca at Jackson Falls, the 100-foot cliffs of Indian Kitchen at Lusk Creek Canyon, and Millstone Bluff, with its fascinating remains of a Woodland and Mississippian Indian settlement. And there's more! Get a trail map or Susan Post's *Hiking Illinois*, mentioned in Appendix B, and explore.

Bell Smith Springs Recreation Area: Red Bud Campground

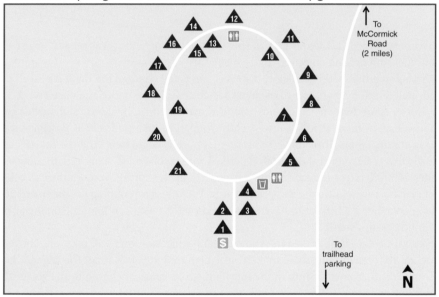

GETTING THERE

From US 45, turn east onto CR 8 (Ozark Road), which will become McCormick Road, and watch for Bell Smith Springs signs. Drive 8.5 miles, turn right at the sign, go 1.6 miles, turn right at the next sign, then continue 2 miles to the campground entrance, on the left.

GPS COORDINATES: N37° 31.136'   W88° 39.348'

30

Camp Cadiz Campground

Beauty ★★★ Privacy ★★★ Spaciousness ★★★ Quiet ★★★★★ Security ★★★ Cleanliness ★★★★

If you're seeking solitude, Camp Cadiz is a good choice.

The eastern Shawnee National Forest boasts some great places for tent campers. Pharaoh Campground at Garden of the Gods is well known for its scenery, Pine Ridge for its beach, and Red Bud for the canyons and streams of nearby Bell Smith Springs.

The Shawnee's easternmost campground, Camp Cadiz, can't offer any of that. What it does offer, however, is your best chance in the whole Shawnee Forest to camp at an established campground with no one else around. If you're seeking solitude but still like the convenience of your car, a toilet, and water nearby, Camp Cadiz is a good choice just about any time outside deer-hunting season. You may, on occasion, find a neighbor or two camping, but chances are they'll be just as eager for quiet as you are.

As you come down Cadiz Road, watch for the old chimneys on the left, the last remnants of the Civilian Conservation Corps camp that once stood here. Turn left, and you'll find the signboard and self-registration post at the entrance to the campground loop. Going counterclockwise around the loop are sites 1–8, each with a fire ring, picnic table, and lantern pole. Site 1, on the outside of the loop at the first chimney, has no shade and, like sites 3 and 5, is too close to the gravel road. Not much traffic passes here, but you might as well be farthest from it. Sites 2 and 4, inside the loop, are grass-covered and somewhat shaded.

The campsite fireplace is the last remnant of the Civilian Conservation Corps camp that once stood here.

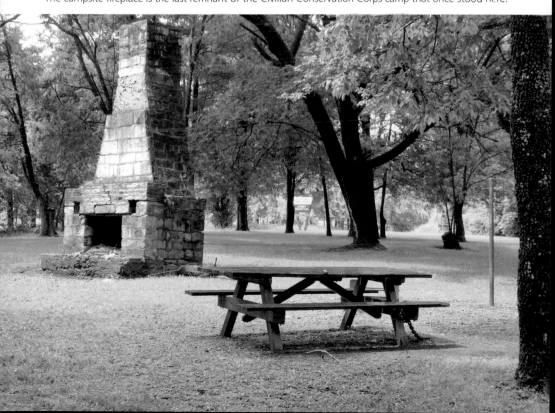

KEY INFORMATION

LOCATION: Cadiz Road, Elizabethtown, IL 62931

CONTACT: Hidden Springs Ranger District, 618-658-2111, bit.ly/CampCadizIL

OPERATED BY: U.S. Forest Service

OPEN: Year-round

SITES: 8 tent sites

EACH SITE HAS: Picnic table, fire ring, and lantern pole

WHEELCHAIR ACCESS: Restrooms and at least one accessible tent site

ASSIGNMENT: First come, first served

REGISTRATION: Register at the self-registration post at the entrance

AMENITIES: Vault toilets, water spigot

PARKING: At site

FEE: $10/night

ELEVATION: 599'

RESTRICTIONS:

PETS: On leash only

QUIET HOURS: 10 p.m.–6 a.m.

FIRES: In fire rings only

ALCOHOL: Permitted

VEHICLES: 2 per site

OTHER: 14-day limit; 2 tents and 8 campers per site

Sites 6 and 7 are by the water spigot. The best site is 8 because it's at the edge of the woods. Note that you may rarely see equestrians camping here.

When I was at Camp Cadiz, the water spigot was broken (it was fixed later in the season), and some sites needed mowing. Forest Service personnel keep up with maintenance as best they can, but the Shawnee is vast. Some repairs and even routine upkeep can be delayed, particularly at a little-visited site like Camp Cadiz. This is one campground where you'd be wise to bring drinking water and even toilet paper, just in case. You can also check the Shawnee National Forest's homepage before coming (www.fs.usda.gov/shawnee), where you'll find regularly updated information about closings and changes in available services.

Camp Cadiz is a trailhead for the River-to-River Trail, which runs approximately 160 miles (or more, depending on who's measuring) across southern Illinois, from Battery Rock on the Ohio River in the east to Devil's Backbone on the Mississippi to the west. Backpackers who use Camp Cadiz as a starting point can park on the grass opposite sites 6 and 7. If you're not up to the whole multiweek trek, there are, fortunately, more than 20 trailheads along it where you can park and day hike specific sections. If you have a hiking partner with a second vehicle, you can shuttle one to your destination, hike, and return in comfort to your campsite, perhaps stopping for a well-earned dinner on the way. From Camp Cadiz you can go south to Rock Creek (about 4 miles), or north to High Knob (about 10 miles—a popular and scenic stretch). Note that you may be sharing the trail with horses and mountain bikers. The River-to-River is generally well blazed—its sign bearing a blue lowercase "i" in a white diamond—but if you plan to hike any portion, you should definitely invest in a topographical map and a compass or GPS. You can find trail maps on the national forest website (www.fs.usda.gov/main/shawnee/maps-pubs), and the Friends of the Shawnee sell excellent maps of the area (shawneefriends.org).

Many visitors to the area hit Garden of the Gods and conclude they've "done" the Shawnee, but whether you hike or drive, go to High Knob, which boasts its own spectacular and less-seen views and rock formations. This rocky prominence sits at 929 feet, with about 2 miles of loop trail circling the base of the cliffs, passing shelter bluffs and traversing slot canyons. Head east on Cadiz Road to Karbers Ridge Road, 5.3 miles from Camp Cadiz. Turn right at the High Knob sign, go 1.7 miles north, and turn right again to reach the parking area. A short trail leads to an overlook; the loop trails begin back down the road a bit.

Not far south or east of Camp Cadiz, you'll find the Ohio River, with its interesting small towns and scenic overlooks. Historic Battery Rock was so named because it served as a fortification during the Civil War. Guns were mounted in the square holes in the rocks, and if you look carefully you'll see names and the date 1861 engraved in the stone. To get there from Camp Cadiz, head east on Cadiz Road to IL 1. Turn right and drive 6.4 miles south to Lamb Road. Turn left and proceed 5.7 miles, going straight at the fork at 4.5 miles, and left at the fork at 5.4 miles.

Camp Cadiz Campground

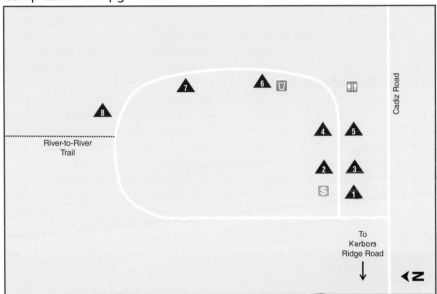

GETTING THERE

From Harrisburg, take IL 34 south 15.3 miles to Karbers Ridge Road. Turn left and go 9.6 miles east to Camp Cadiz entrance on the left.

From the junction of IL 1 and IL 13, go 12.5 miles south on IL 1 to Cadiz Road. Turn right and go 2.8 miles west to Camp Cadiz entrance on the right.

GPS COORDINATES: N37° 34.651'   W88° 14.699'

31

Cave-in-Rock State Park

Beauty ★★★ Privacy ★★★ Spaciousness ★★★ Quiet ★★★ Security ★★★★★ Cleanliness ★★★★

Take in the sweeping views of the Ohio River valley from this historic—and even notorious—landmark.

Few parks in Illinois can lay claim to as much fascinating history and even notoriety as Cave-in-Rock State Park, just east of the town of the same name on the Ohio River. From the 1790s to the 1830s, the 55-foot-wide cave in a bluff overlooking the river served variously as a hideout for counterfeiters, a lair for pirates who preyed on river traffic, and a "Liquor Vault and House of Entertainment." The cave itself is equally intriguing, and this is one place in southern Illinois where you're sure to see flocks of tourists during the summer. Fortunately, most don't spend the night, so the campground, while popular, is not nearly so crowded.

As you enter the park, take the first left. You'll enter the Class A section of the campground, a large loop of 34 electric sites with plenty of grassy space but not much shade. Many sites have ample room for tents, but RVs predominate, and most weekends this area will be at least three-quarters full. Continue right around the circle, and take the next right uphill to the entrance to the tent-camping area. Sixteen nonelectric sites lie along two spurs: sites 1–6 are on the left, and 7–16 are on the right. All sites have a ground grill and table; there are water and vault toilets at the tent-area entrance. Additionally, all campers can use the shower house in the Class A section. Sites here are smaller but better shaded, and this area isn't as busy—perhaps half full on nonholiday weekends.

The spur to the left is on sloping ground, so I prefer the more level sites to the right. Sites 11, 13, and 14 are nicely shaded, and 16 is a bit farther from the road and other sites.

Cave-in-Rock, as seen from the Ohio River   *photo by W Eugene Slowik*

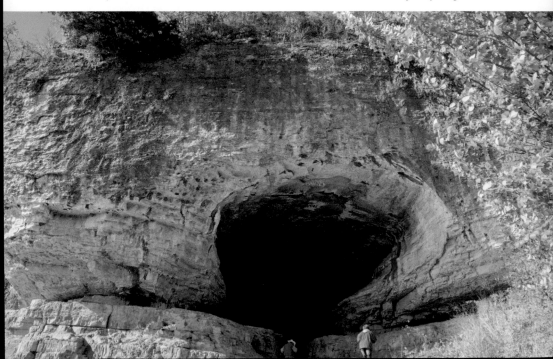

KEY INFORMATION

LOCATION: #1 New State Park Road, Box 338, Cave-In-Rock, IL 62919

CONTACT: 618-289-4325, bit.ly/CaveInRockIL

OPERATED BY: IDNR

OPEN: Year-round

SITES: 34 Class A sites; 16 Class B sites

EACH SITE HAS: Picnic table, fire ring and grate; electricity (Class A only)

WHEELCHAIR ACCESS: Restrooms and at least one accessible tent site

ASSIGNMENT: First come, first served

REGISTRATION: Register with the host or set up and park staff will come by

AMENITIES: Water spigots, vault toilets, shower house; lodge with 4 duplex cottages; restaurant

PARKING: At site

FEE: Class A: $20/night, $30/night holidays; Class B: $10/night

ELEVATION: 344'

RESTRICTIONS:

PETS: On leash only

QUIET HOURS: 10 p.m.–7 a.m.

FIRES: In fire rings only

ALCOHOL: Permitted

VEHICLES: 4 per site

OTHER: 14-day limit; 1 RV and 1 tent, or 4 tents per site

You can go ahead and set up before registering with the campground host at site 1 in the Class A section, or park staff will come by later. Firewood is usually available from the campground host.

For those not wanting to rough it, Cave-in-Rock also has four duplex cabins with eight suites altogether. Each suite has two queen beds, a living room, a private bathroom, a refrigerator, microwave, coffee maker, and a private deck with unrivaled views of the Ohio River. The small restaurant offers a good selection of breakfast items, sandwiches, and dinners, including an all-you-can-eat catfish and fried chicken buffet on Sundays. The restaurant is open April–October, daily except for Tuesday. Call 618-289-4545 or check caveinrockkaylors.com for more information.

You'll, of course, want to see the cave: the short trail begins at the parking area across the road from the campground entrance. Be careful—as you descend the rough stone steps, you'll want to take in the sweeping views of the Ohio River, almost 0.5 mile wide at this point. Although the cave entrance is huge, the cave itself is only about 160 feet deep. A sinkhole in the ceiling forms a natural skylight, so you won't need a flashlight. This is a cool place on a hot summer day. Unlike the sandstone bluff shelters in the Shawnee Forest, this is a solutional cave, formed as water pushed its way out to the river, gradually dissolving the limestone bedrock. At one time the cave was probably much longer, but over thousands of years the Ohio River shaved off its southern end.

Most visitors "do" the cave and then leave, missing the hiking trails and opportunities to explore the woods and the park's scenic vistas. Make the most of this park: You can pick up the Hickory Ridge and Pirate's Bluff Trails east of the tent campground; together they total about 1.75 miles. There are other unmarked trails along the river and bluffs.

About 4 miles west of the town of Cave-in-Rock, you can get another outstanding view of the river valley from the bluffs at Tower Rock. Head west on Clay Street, which becomes Cave-in-Rock Road, to Tower Rock Road, and turn left. A short trail from the east side of the parking area climbs to the overlook. You can also camp here (no fee, no facilities), but the area is sometimes closed due to flooding. Call the U.S. Forest Service at 618-658-2111 for current information.

For a different view of the Ohio River, take the free ferry across to Kentucky. You can drive or even just walk from the park entrance to the crossing on Canal Street (Route 1). The ferry runs daily, 6 a.m.–9:45 p.m.

If you want to scope out the diverse flora and fauna of the region, check out any of the trails at the War Bluff Valley Sanctuary, managed by the Shawnee Chapter of the Illinois Audubon Society. At almost 500 acres, War Bluff is the largest Audubon sanctuary in the state, and home to a wide variety of birds, mammals, reptiles, and amphibians. You'll find several miles of maintained trails winding among seven ponds, a clear creek, historic homestead sites, and limestone outcroppings. From Cave-in-Rock, take IL 1 north to IL 146, turn left, and go 21 miles to Bushwhack Road. Turn right, and continue 2.25 miles to the sanctuary entrance on the right. Check shawneeaudubon.wordpress.com or call 618-683-2222.

Cave-in-Rock State Park: Tent Area

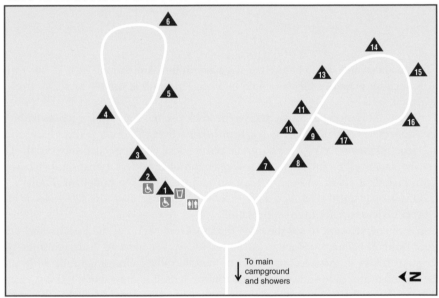

GETTING THERE

From I-57 at Marion, take Exit 54 to access IL 13 East. Go 38 miles, through Harrisburg, to IL 1. Turn right and drive 22 miles south to the town of Cave-in-Rock. Turn left at the park sign on Main Street, and head 0.25 mile to the park entrance.

GPS COORDINATES: N37° 28.042'   W88° 09.733'

32

Devils Kitchen Campground

Beauty ★★★★ Privacy ★★★ Spaciousness ★★★ Quiet ★★★★ Security ★★★★★ Cleanliness ★★★★★

Unique to Devils Kitchen Campground are the individual boat slips, one for each campsite.

The campground at Devils Kitchen Lake has been around for a while—but it is also new. It was formerly a 45-site RV campground privately operated under license from the U.S. Department of Fish & Wildlife, which owns the almost 44,000 acres of Crab Orchard National Wildlife Refuge in which the campground is located. In 2006, however, Fish & Wildlife decided to assume direct management and return the area to a more primitive state, allowing only tent camping. It reopened in 2009 as a small, quiet campground surrounded by rocky outcroppings on a scenic, tree-lined lake.

The signboard at the entrance to Devils Kitchen Campground is where you self-register after selecting your site. To use any of the facilities within the refuge (lakes, boat ramps, parking areas, or trails), you also need a vehicle pass, which you can purchase here.

The wood-encircled camping area is on a large grass-covered point that juts into the northern end of Devils Kitchen Lake. Eight primitive walk-in sites form a circle around the clearing, and cedar posts and railings border each site, which has its own table, ground grill, and lantern post. The closest wheelchair-accessible site is by the parking lot; the farthest is about 250 feet away. The sites are fairly far apart and have some shade, though there's not much brush separating them. If all eight were occupied, it might feel busy, but with so few sites, this should still be a quiet spot. You'll find a water spigot in the middle of the campground, and the shower house and restrooms are just across the parking lot.

Sunset on Devils Kitchen Lake

photo by Pete Dunkel

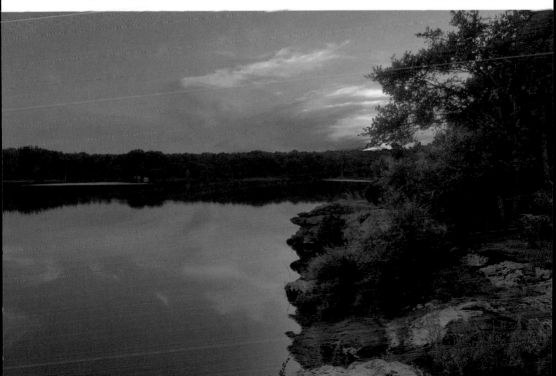

KEY INFORMATION

LOCATION: Tacoma Lake Road, Makanda, IL, 62958

CONTACT: Crab Orchard office: 618-997-3344, fws.gov/midwest/craborchard (no specific campground website)

OPERATED BY: Crab Orchard National Wildlife Refuge, U.S. Department of Fish & Wildlife

OPEN: April 1–October 31

SITES: 8 walk-in tent sites

EACH SITE HAS: Picnic table, fire ring, lantern post

WHEELCHAIR ACCESS: Restrooms and at least one accessible tent site

ASSIGNMENT: First come, first served

REGISTRATION: Register at the self-registration post at the entrance

AMENITIES: Water spigot, shower house with flush toilets, boat slips

PARKING: In lot

FEE: $10/night

ELEVATION: 545'

RESTRICTIONS:

PETS: On leash only

QUIET HOURS: 11 p.m.–7 a.m.

FIRES: In fire rings only

ALCOHOL: Not permitted

VEHICLES: 2 per site

OTHER: 14-day limit; 8 people per site

Wildlife is abundant around Devils Kitchen. You may see a beaver swimming by in the evening, deer by the restrooms, or a family of raccoons near the campground. The refuge as a whole is home to more than 260 bird species, including some nesting pairs of bald eagles.

Unique to Devils Kitchen Campground are the individual boat docks, one for each campsite. Take the short trail down from the parking area to the little inlet, where you'll find eight beautiful wooden boat slips. The campground is primitive, but the boat slips have lights and electrical hookups. The boat ramp is down the road just before the campground entrance. Note that boats using the lake must have a pass, available from the refuge visitor center on IL 148 in Carbondale or from the marina at Little Grassy Lake. Boats on Devils Kitchen must be 10 horsepower or less.

Though small, the campground is usually only about half full on nonholiday weekends. With various other camping options nearby (Giant City, Little Grassy, Crab Orchard), Devils Kitchen is relatively unnoticed.

All three of the refuge lakes are popular for boating and fishing. Crab Orchard is the largest lake, at 6,900 acres, and is busy with sailboats and water-skiers on warm summer days. Crappie and largemouth bass fishing here are excellent. On the northwest end, just off Spillway Road, south of IL 13, there's a full-service marina where you can rent boats. The 1,200-acre Little Grassy Lake, to the west of Devils Kitchen, is quieter and also has a marina and a small beach. Devils Kitchen covers 810 acres and has been intentionally left the least developed. With a maximum depth of 90 feet, it is also the second-deepest lake in Illinois (surpassed only by Lake Michigan), and the crystal-clear, cool waters are ideal for rainbow trout. This is one of the few places in southern Illinois where you can fish for trout year-round. For more details and a map of all the refuge lakes and ponds, pick up the Crab Orchard fishing brochure at the campground signboard.

Three of the refuge's five established hiking trails are located around Devils Kitchen Lake. If you have time for just one, take the 1.8-mile Rocky Bluff Trail. The trailhead is about 0.5 mile south of the campground, on Tacoma Lake Road (there is parking on the left). This moderately difficult loop will take you through sandstone canyons and past seasonal waterfalls and shelter caves. It is especially beautiful (and popular) in the spring, when wildflowers of all colors carpet the canyon floor. Note that the trail can be muddy and the wet sandstone slippery.

Offering scenic views of Devils Kitchen Lake, Grassy Creek Trail is a 1.4-mile loop with a wide, paved surface that was once an old road. To get to the trail parking, head south on Tacoma Lake Road about 2.9 miles from the campground, then turn right and drive 0.5 mile just over Grassy Creek Bridge. Maps and descriptions of all the trails are available online (bit.ly/CrabOrchardTrails) or at the refuge visitor center, where you can pick up a printed guide for the 9-mile auto tour of the refuge as well. Check their Facebook page (facebook .com/CrabOrchardNWR) for a variety of special programs, including auto, biking, kayak, and birding tours, some of which go into areas of the refuge not otherwise open to the public. All are free, but some require advance registration.

Devils Kitchen Campground

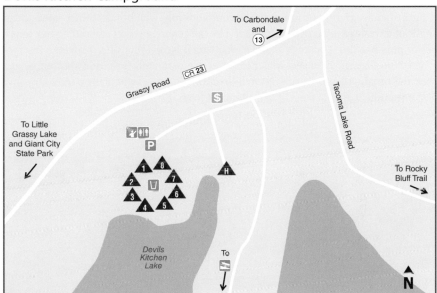

GETTING THERE

From I-57, take Exit 54 in Marion, go west 10.2 miles on IL 13, and make the first left after crossing Crab Orchard Lake onto Spillway Road. Follow Spillway Road 9 miles (it joins Grassy Road at 8 miles) to Tacoma Lake Road. Turn left, then make the first right into the campground.

From US 51 and IL 13 in Carbondale, go 4.1 miles east to Spillway Road, turn right, go 9 miles south, and proceed as above at Tacoma Lake Road.

GPS COORDINATES: N37° 38.794' W89° 06.287'

33

⛺ Dixon Springs State Park

Beauty ★★★★★ Privacy ★★★★ Spaciousness ★★★ Quiet ★★★★ Security ★★★★ Cleanliness ★★★★

If the kids want to do something other than just enjoy nature, you have great options at Dixon Springs.

Dixon Springs has long been a place to welcome visitors. More than a century ago, there was a small community, with a post office, gristmill, and general store here. Later a resort developed, complete with a hotel and cabins, and people came from Illinois and neighboring states to take advantage of the purported medicinal benefits of the seven springs for which the town was named. The springs are no longer a prime attraction, but the park and surrounding area still offer lots to see and do, along with a separate, peaceful tent-camping area.

As you enter Dixon Springs off IL 146, go straight, make the second right, and head up the hill, following the signs for tent camping. The road turns right at three historic church buildings and then comes to a picnic pavilion, where you'll find parking for the walk-in tent area. Park staff are rightly proud of this recent addition, which has 10 nice sites scattered throughout a wooded area. Most are shaded by tall pines, and you can pitch your tent on a carpet of pine needles. Unlike at many parks, which have a few sites dispersed in an open area, at Dixon Springs at least some of the sites are separated from one another by stands of trees and brush. All are considered walk-in sites, but you can actually park your car right next to site 1; site 9, the farthest, is only 215 feet from the lot.

Stone and water characterize the scenic terrain at Dixon Springs.

photo by J. M. Hagstrom

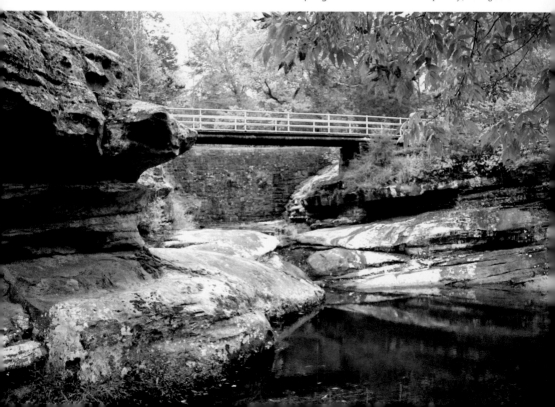

KEY INFORMATION

LOCATION: 24 Park Road, Golconda, IL 62938

CONTACT: 618-949-3394,
bit.ly/DixonSprings-IL

OPERATED BY: IDNR

OPEN: Year-round

SITES: Class B: 39 sites; Class D: 10 walk-in
tent sites

EACH SITE HAS: Picnic table, fire ring;
only Class B has electricity

WHEELCHAIR ACCESS: Restrooms and at
least one accessible electric site

ASSIGNMENT: First come, first served;
reservations available online

REGISTRATION: Set up and park staff will
come by

AMENITIES: Water spigots, vault toilets;
swimming pool available for fee

PARKING: Class B: at site; Class D: in lot

FEE: Class B: $18/night; Class D: $6/night

ELEVATION: 507'

RESTRICTIONS:

PETS: On leash only

QUIET HOURS: 10 p.m.–7 a.m.

FIRES: In fire rings only

ALCOHOL: Permitted

VEHICLES: 2 per site

OTHER: 14-day limit; 1 RV and 1 tent,
or 2 tents per site; 4 adults or 1 family
per site

Just off the parking lot, to the right, you'll see a trail with a yellow gate that allows walk-in access to most of the sites. The ones to the left of the trail (sites 1–8) are under pine trees. Site 5 is my favorite because it's set back from the others and surrounded by trees so you won't be disturbed by other campers hiking through or around your campsite to reach theirs. Sites 9 and 10 are in deciduous woods; 9 is especially private. Sites 1–4 are close to parking—great, as long as you're not sharing the campground with too many other parties. And more often than not, you won't be. On an average nonholiday weekend, only three or four sites will be occupied.

Unless you've reserved a site online, pick an unreserved site and set up. Park staff will come by to register you. You'll find vault toilets beyond the campsites and a water spigot and toilets next to the pavilion by the parking lot. The showers are by the swimming pool—check with the park staff or the campground host in the RV section for information. If you want electricity, there is a separate Class B campground with 39 sites. For groups of up to 80 people, there are six dorm cabins with a kitchen and shower house that can be reserved online through reserveamerica.com.

If you've ever taken kids camping and found they want to *do* something rather than just sit around and enjoy nature, you've got some great options at Dixon Springs. They will love the pool with the 45-foot water slide and wading pool for the little ones, and there's a snack bar with sweets and sandwiches. It's open Memorial Day–mid-August, daily, 11:30 a.m.–5:30 p.m. It costs $5 for the whole day, and is free for kids under age 3. A private concessionaire operates the pool; call 618-949-3871 for current information.

Before swimming, you and the kids can get a little nature in with a hike on Ghost Dance Canyon Trail, which starts right by the pool parking lot. The name alone is sure to pique their interest, and the canyon will hold it. The trail winds between canyon walls as high as 60 feet, following a rippling creek past a waterfall and huge stands of boulders that beg to be explored. The trail itself is 1 mile long, but the canyon continues, and you can push farther without fear of getting lost. Bring a camera—you'll want to get photos of some of the unique rock formations and perhaps a shot of the kids perched atop a mound of boulders like conquering heroes.

Just 3 miles north of Dixon Springs, on IL 145, is Lake Glendale (lakeglendale.net), with boating, fishing, and a public beach. And if you have an archaeological bent, head 5 miles farther north to Millstone Bluff (bit.ly/MillstoneBluff), the remains of a prehistoric Woodland and Mississippian Indian settlement perched on a cliff rising 320 feet above the surrounding terrain. A 0.5-mile trail takes you past the remains of the cemetery and a village that was probably last occupied around 1500 A.D. There isn't a lot to see, but you may find it fascinating, as I do, to read the interpretive signs and imagine those who lived there some 500 years ago. Head north on IL 145—just east of the park—and drive 5.5 miles to IL 147. Turn left (west), and go 1 mile to the entrance to Millstone Bluff, on the right.

And at least stop and be tempted by the amazing array of confections just across the highway from the park at the Chocolate Factory. Open Monday through Saturday, they also have fountain drinks and ice cream. Check thechocolatefactory.net for more information.

GETTING THERE

From I-24, take Exit 16 at Vienna to access IL 146 East. Go 12 miles to the park entrance, on the left.

GPS COORDINATES: N37° 22.826'   W88° 39.964'

Dixon Springs State Park

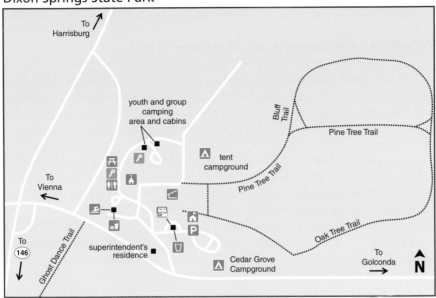

Dixon Springs State Park: Tent Campground

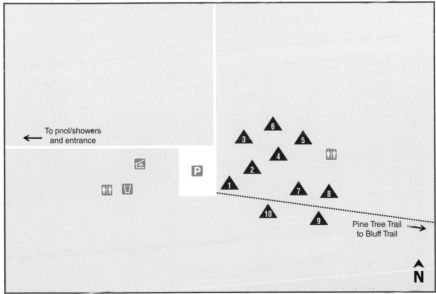

Ferne Clyffe State Park

Beauty ★★★★★ Privacy ★★★★ Spaciousness ★★★★★ Quiet ★★★★★ Security ★★★★ Cleanliness ★★★★★

Ferne Clyffe is a hiker's paradise, with 18 well-marked trails.

Before I ever contemplated writing this book, Ferne Clyffe was my favorite place to camp in Illinois. I'm now finishing the second edition, and it still is. The combination of beautiful, secluded, comfortable campsites and excellent hiking draws me back again and again. Since it's right in the middle of southern Illinois, it's also a great base from which to explore the Shawnee Forest.

Enter the park off IL 37 and go 0.5 mile to the stop sign. Uphill and straight ahead is the RV campground—turn left instead. At the Y-intersection by the lake, you may be sorely tempted to stop and take in the tranquil view—save that for later. Take the left fork and follow the signs to Turkey Ridge tent camping (turn right, then left).

A tent camper must have designed this campground. Each of the 20 sites is a short walk from parking, yet most of them are surrounded by enough trees and brush to make you feel like you're all alone. All are beautifully shaded, and many are on raised flat pads bordered by landscaping timbers. Each has a ground grill, table, and lantern post, and all campers can use the main campground's shower building (closed late November–April 1).

My favorite site is 10: all the way at the end, it is large, flat, and well secluded from its only neighbor, site 9. Because it's on a hill below the level of the parking lot, you can't see the lot from the site. Sites 1–9 are tucked away in the woods, accessed by short trails—

Tent campsite at Turkey Ridge

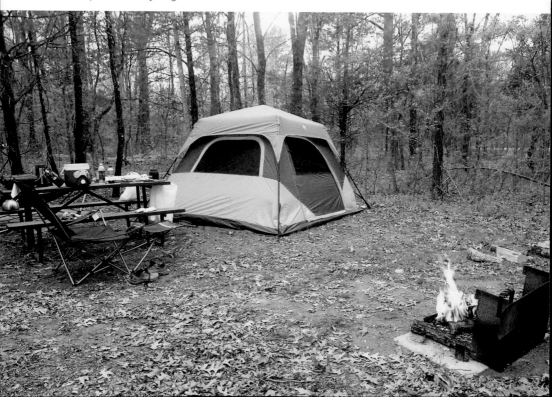

KEY INFORMATION

LOCATION: 8235 S. Broadway, Goreville, IL 62939

CONTACT: 618-995-2411, bit.ly/FerneClyffeIL

OPERATED BY: IDNR

OPEN: Year-round (backpacking sites closed third weekend in November to first weekend in December)

SITES: Class A: 59 sites (Deer Ridge); Class B: 20 walk-in (Turkey Ridge); 3 backpacking sites

EACH SITE HAS: Picnic table, fire ring; electricity (Class A only)

WHEELCHAIR ACCESS: Restrooms and at least one accessible electric site

ASSIGNMENT: First come, first served; reservations available online (Class A only)

REGISTRATION: Register with the host in Deer Ridge or set up and park staff will come by

AMENITIES: Flush toilets, showers (Deer Ridge, available to all), water spigots, vault toilets

PARKING: At site (Deer Ridge); in lot (Turkey Ridge and backpacking sites)

FEE: Deer Ridge: $20/night, $30/night on holidays; all others: $8/night

ELEVATION: 712'

RESTRICTIONS:

PETS: On leash only

QUIET HOURS: 10 p.m.–7 a.m.

FIRES: In fire rings only

ALCOHOL: Permitted

VEHICLES: 2 per site

OTHER: 14-day limit; 1 RV and 1 tent, or 2 tents per site; 4 adults or 1 family per site

---

1 is probably the best of these, as long as there's no one at nearby site 2. Sites 11 and 12 are attractive and spacious but a bit close to parking for me. Sites 13–18 are all in the woods, off a short half-circle trail. Watch for poison ivy—it abounds off the trails around sites 1–10.

If Turkey Ridge is full (possible on weekends), or if you'd like more privacy, there are three backpacking sites. You can take the backpack trail at the end of the parking lot for a hilly 0.75-mile hike—a bit of work if you're hauling stuff. There's a simple shortcut: go between sites 1 and 2, cut across a short bit of woods until you reach an obvious trail, and turn left. You've just bypassed the hilly part, and now it's only 0.2 level miles to the backpack sites. These sites are in the woods and each has a fire ring and table.

Ferne Clyffe is a hiker's paradise. There are 18 well-marked hiking trails, ranging from 0.25 to 8 miles in length, which take you along high sandstone bluffs, through cool canyons, and by seasonal waterfalls and shelter bluff caves. Many of the trails connect, and it's helpful to have the map and trail descriptions handy; find them on the park website or in the brochure. Many of the most popular trails can be accessed from the parking loop at the end of the picnic shelter road—take the right fork at the Y-intersection by the lake. Some of the "ooh-ahh" sights are actually not too far from here—nice if you have kids who aren't up for a long trek. Hawk's Cave Trail is an easy 0.5-mile loop leading to a 150-foot sandstone cave, and a 100-foot seasonal waterfall is an easy 0.75-mile round-trip via Big Rocky Hollow Trail.

Rock climbing and rappelling are permitted in two areas of the park: off Rebman Trail and at Cedar Bluff. No permission is required—climb at your own risk, and be sure you know what you're doing. And if you don't know what you're doing but would like to learn, check out Vertical Heartland, just 8 miles southwest of Ferne Clyffe. At this privately owned portion of Draper's Bluff, Eric Ulner offers half-day and full-day climbing instruction for individuals, families, and groups—no experience is required. Call 618-995-1427 for a reservation, or check verticalheartland.com for more information.

South of Ferne Clyffe is the unique Cache River State Natural Area, almost 15,000 acres of wetlands that look like Louisiana bayous. You can explore trails and boardwalks over the swamp—don't miss the state's oldest living resident, a bald cypress tree that's more than 1,000 years old. Start at the excellent Barkhausen Wetlands Visitor Center, 16.5 miles south of the Ferne Clyffe entrance on IL 37, open Wednesday–Sunday, 9 a.m.–4 p.m. Call 618-657-2064 for information. There is also a fascinating, well-marked canoe trail through the lower Cache River. To really experience the Cache with people who know it well, contact White Crane Canoe Rentals & Guide Service. They can set you up with kayaks or canoes and laminated trail maps, or take you on a very informative guided trip. Call 618-201-4090 or check whitecranecanoes.com for more information.

Cycling is popular on nearby Tunnel Hill Trail, a 45-mile hike-and-bike trail built along abandoned railroad beds. There are numerous access points, but the 9.3-mile section from Tunnel Hill to Vienna is perhaps the most scenic and has several unique features, including the 543-foot tunnel and the longest and highest trestle on the trail. From Ferne Clyffe, go 0.5 mile north on IL 37 to Tunnel Hill Road, then drive 8 miles east. Check bit.ly/TunnelHill-IL or call 618-658-2168 for more information.

GETTING THERE

From I-57, take Exit 40 east, then go 4 miles on CR 13 to Goreville. Turn right on IL 37 and follow it 1.5 miles south to the park entrance, on the left.

From I-24, take Exit 7 west to IL 37 in Goreville and turn left. Go 1.5 miles south to the park entrance, on the left.

GPS COORDINATES: N37° 31.944'   W88° 57.973'

Bork Falls is accessible via a short trail.

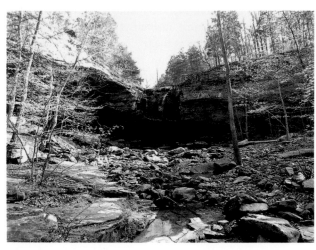

Ferne Clyffe State Park

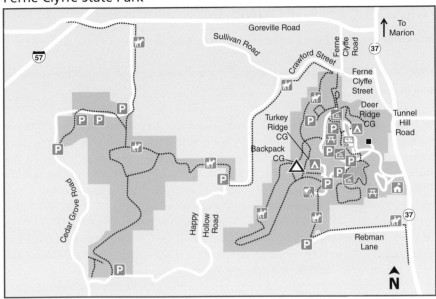

Ferne Clyffe State Park: Turkey Ridge Campground

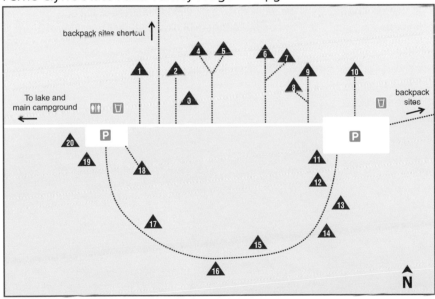

35

Garden of the Gods Recreation Area:
PHARAOH CAMPGROUND

Beauty ★★★★★ Privacy ★★★ Spaciousness ★★★ Quiet ★★★★★ Security ★★★★ Cleanliness ★★★★

Pharaoh Campground is a popular but quiet retreat amid some of the most spectacular scenery in Illinois.

Pharaoh Campground at Garden of the Gods Recreation Area is a popular but quiet retreat amid some of the most spectacular scenery in Illinois. Whether you camp there or just visit for the day while staying elsewhere, Garden of the Gods is a must-see.

The drive to Garden of the Gods is almost as beautiful as the destination itself. It is located along Karbers Ridge Road, which snakes among wooded hills and rolling meadows as it passes through the Shawnee National Forest. Whether you pick up Karbers Ridge off IL 1 to the east or IL 34 to the west, take your time and enjoy the scenery.

Turn north off Karbers Ridge Road at the Garden of the Gods sign, and go about 1.4 miles to the left turn into the recreation area. Another 1.4 miles brings you to a T-intersection—take a left for trailhead parking, or a right for the campground.

Pharaoh Campground consists of a single loop with 12 sites on its south side. Each has a fire ring, picnic table, and lantern pole. There's a set of vault toilets next to site 6, and a hand-operated water pump at the loop entrance. Most sites enjoy the shade of tall, stately pines, and some offer a panoramic view of the valley below and the Shawnee Hills. Sites 2 and 10 are well shaded, and 12 offers the most space and seclusion, being at the end. Sites 7 and 9 have the best views, and site 7 has trees on either side, separating it from the adjacent sites.

Overlooking iconic Camel Rock, along the Observation Trail

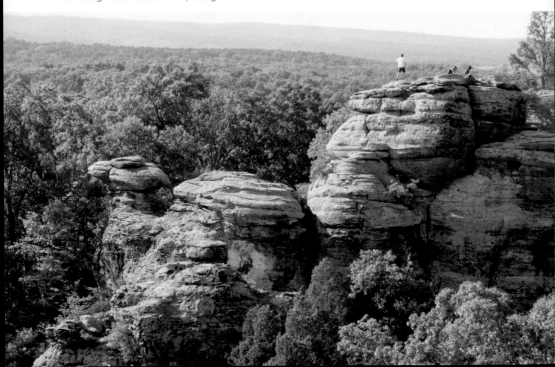

KEY INFORMATION

LOCATION: Garden of the Gods Road, Herod, IL 62947

CONTACT: Hidden Springs Ranger District, 618-658-2111, bit.ly/PharaohIL

OPERATED BY: U.S. Forest Service

OPEN: Year-round

SITES: 12 tent sites

EACH SITE HAS: Picnic table, fire ring, and lantern pole

WHEELCHAIR ACCESS: Restrooms and at least one accessible tent site

ASSIGNMENT: First come, first served

REGISTRATION: Register at the self-registration post at the entrance

AMENITIES: Hand pump, vault toilets

PARKING: At site

FEE: $10/night

ELEVATION: 845'

RESTRICTIONS:

PETS: On leash only

QUIET HOURS: 10 p.m.–6 a.m.

FIRES: In fire rings only

ALCOHOL: Permitted

VEHICLES: 2 per site

OTHER: 14-day limit; 8 campers per site

The most impressive thing about Pharaoh is the quiet. Even some of the most secluded campgrounds I've visited are often close enough to a highway, railway, or just the road through the park that some mechanized noise is inevitable. Not so here. Pharaoh is in the middle of a wilderness area, perched high above the valley, far from any transportation clamor. To be sure, the trailhead parking down on the other side of the T-intersection is very busy, especially on weekends. Garden of the Gods is the most-visited site in the Shawnee National Forest. But that doesn't affect the campground. And though the campground will be nearly full on most fair-weather weekends, the people who camp at Pharaoh are not usually partiers but hikers and backpackers who appreciate and guard the stillness.

If you are fortunate enough to have a clear sky at night at Pharaoh, you can enjoy stargazing as well. With the relatively high altitude (830 feet) and the lack of city lights nearby, the nighttime celestial vistas are as stunning as the daytime terrestrial ones.

At some point during your stay at Pharaoh, you will hike the 0.25-mile Observation Trail. Stroll down the hill to the parking area and trail entrance. Bring drinking water in a nondisposable container (disposables are not permitted). The trail is paved but steep in places, and you'll want good hiking shoes so you can safely clamber up, over, and around these amazing sandstone formations. Be careful near the bluffs and hang on to small children. The sign at the trailhead says to allow 45 minutes, but you may want to spend much longer simply sitting and enjoying the breathtaking views. Bring a camera to snap a picture of Camel Rock, probably the most-photographed natural feature in Illinois.

To see more of the geological wonders of the area, take the trailhead starting at the north end of the parking area. Go 0.2 mile north to the trail junction on the left past Anvil Rock. Turn left (west), and at the next trail junction you can go right (north) or left (south). Going right about 0.5 mile takes you first to Mushroom Rock, and then to the Noah's Ark formation. Head left to pass Shelter Rock and other formations. At 0.6 mile you'll reach the River-to-River Trail. Here take the trail marked "Lower Trail." You pass beneath all the formations seen from the Observation Trail. After 0.5 mile you'll cross the park road. Follow the trail as it circles the bluffs below the camping area. At 0.75 mile from the road, you'll reach another trail junction on the left. Make the left and climb 0.25 mile to the campground road. These trails are normally well signed, but it's wise to bring a trail map just in case. A useful one can be found at bit.ly/GoGTrailMap.

If you want to visit Garden of the Gods but would rather camp some place less busy, try Camp Cadiz—head 3 miles east on Karbers Ridge Road, take a right on Cadiz Road, then go 3.7 miles. If you'd like a campground with a swimming beach, check out Pine Ridge at the Pounds Hollow Recreation Area, 6.6 miles east on Karbers Ridge Road.

Garden of the Gods Recreation Area: Pharaoh Campground

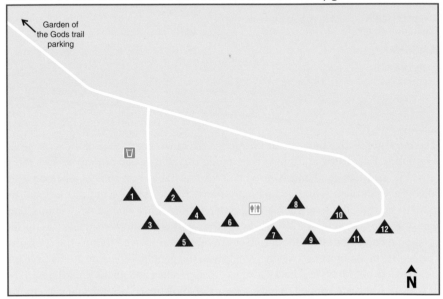

GETTING THERE

From Harrisburg, take IL 34 south 15.3 miles to Karbers Ridge Road. Turn left and go 2.8 miles to the Garden of the Gods sign at CR 10. Make another left and proceed 1.4 miles north to the entrance, on the left.

From IL 1, turn west onto CR 13/Pounds Hollow Road. Go 8.5 miles (this becomes Karbers Ridge Road) to the sign at CR 10, turn right, and drive 1.4 miles north to the entrance, on the left.

GPS COORDINATES: N37° 36.235'   W88° 23.004'

36

Giant City State Park

Beauty ★★★ Privacy ★★ Spaciousness ★★★ Quiet ★★★ Security ★★★★★ Cleanliness ★★★★★

Do not miss the chance to hike amid the fascinating rock formations that have earned this park its name.

Giant City State Park has something for everyone. Whether you enjoy rappelling, horseback riding, or relaxing in the air-conditioned comfort of a completely furnished cabin, you'll find it here. A prime attraction is the hiking: trek amid the fascinating rock formations that have earned this park its name. Tent campers have their own separate area, and though it can seem crowded on busy weekends, it's well worth it to experience all that this beautiful park has to offer.

If you enter the park from the north on Giant City Road, turn left onto the first road, toward the campground. If entering from Makanda or US 51, take the first left and then the second right onto the campground road. Turn right into the campground, where you'll find the host's site on the right. Pick an unreserved site, set up, and register with the host (if available) or at the self-registration post there.

The 85 Class A electric sites in the main campground are average RV sites. To find a better choice for tent camping, go all the way to the south end of the campground on the middle road to reach the parking area for the walk-in tent-camping sites. There are 14 campsites here—each with a table and ground grill—scattered around a grassy area that is shaded by pine and deciduous trees. These are farther apart than the RV sites, but there still isn't much brush between them—you and your neighbors will have to pretend you have more privacy than you really do.

Explore the avenues between massive stone blocks on the Giant City Trail.   *photo by David Lauchner*

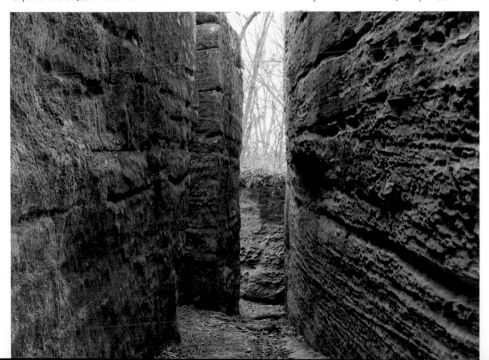

KEY INFORMATION

LOCATION: 235 Giant City Road, Makanda, IL 62958

CONTACT: 618-457-4836, bit.ly/GiantCityIL

OPERATED BY: IDNR

OPEN: Year-round

SITES: Class A: 85 sites; Class C: 14 walk-in sites

EACH SITE HAS: Picnic table, fire ring; electricity (Class A only)

WHEELCHAIR ACCESS: Restrooms and at least one accessible electric site

ASSIGNMENT: First come, first served

REGISTRATION: Register with the campground host (if available) or at the self-registration post

AMENITIES: Water spigots, vault toilets, shower house (closed December 1–April 1)

PARKING: Class A: at site; Class C and backpacking: in lot

FEE: Class A: $20/night, $30/night holidays; Class C and backpacking: $8/night

ELEVATION: 676'

RESTRICTIONS:

PETS: On leash only

QUIET HOURS: 10 p.m.–7 a.m.

FIRES: In fire rings only

ALCOHOL: Permitted in campground only

VEHICLES: 2 per site

OTHER: 14-day limit; 1 RV and 1 tent, or 2 tents per site; 4 adults or 1 family per site

---

And almost any time during the regular camping season you will have neighbors. Giant City is popular, and even the tent sites can fill on fair-weather weekends. For that reason I suggest walking the 200-feet or so to one of the sites farthest from the road—4, 5, 7, 8, or 9. You'll be out of the flow of traffic to the other sites, will have a bit more shade, and still won't feel as crowded as you would in the RV campground—but you can use the same modern shower house. The walk-in sites are all first come, first served, but any of the Class A sites can be reserved online at reserveamerica.com.

Backpackers can try the 12-mile Red Cedar Trail, which has four primitive sites with toilets (but no water) at the 6-mile point on the trail. Register first with the campground host or park office, and park at the trailhead by the walk-in sites. Even here, though, you may not find seclusion on the weekends, since these sites are popular with students from nearby Southern Illinois University.

Do not miss the chance to hike at Giant City. To best appreciate what you'll see, first stop at the visitor center to view the displays and a short film about the geology of the area and pick up the detailed hiking guides for each trail. Kids can explore hands-on exhibits in the Discovery Corner. Then take the 1-mile Giant City Trail, which winds through sandstone blocks left after eons of erosion created what today seem like "avenues" amid the buildings of a city for giants—hence the park's name. Kids love to scramble around these. Other short trails lead past sandstone bluffs, inspiring overlooks, a cool shelter cave, and the remnants of a stone wall left by American Indians. You can download interpretive guides for all park trails from the website.

Even if you enjoy roughing it, spend a few minutes indoors at the rustic and comfortable Giant City Lodge. This building was constructed by the Civilian Conservation Corps in the 1930s from local sandstone and white-oak timbers and has been renovated and expanded, maintaining its historic beauty. To get away from campfire cooking, try their excellent Bald Knob dining room before you leave, taking advantage of their Sunday fried chicken buffet or Friday night catfish buffet—it's usually wise to make reservations on the weekend. Friends or family who'd rather have a bed can rent one of the fully furnished cabins and swim in the pool during the summer. Check giantcitylodge.com or call 618-457-4921 for reservations.

Horseback riding for kids and adults is available through Giant City Stables, a private concession in the park. They offer guided trail rides, lessons, and pony rides for the younger wranglers. You can get more information and current rates at 618-529-4110 or giantcitystables.com.

Rock climbing and rappelling are permitted in two places: at the bluffs by Devil's Standtable and at Shelter #1. No check-in or registration is necessary—just be sure you know what you're doing, bring your own equipment, and understand that you climb at your own risk. You can't install permanent anchors, but the park is working on setting up a few sportclimbing routes.

If you want another hike amid interesting geology, head for Rocky Bluff Trail at nearby Devils Kitchen Lake. From Giant City, go 3 miles north on Giant City Road to Little Grassy Road and turn right. Drive 3.5 miles to Tacoma Lake Road, turn right, and go 0.5 mile to the Rocky Bluff trailhead parking. This 1.8-mile loop will take you past seasonal waterfalls and sandstone cliffs. Devils Kitchen Lake is part of the Crab Orchard National Wildlife Refuge, so a $2-per-day vehicle tag is necessary and can be purchased at one of the refuge campgrounds.

Giant City State Park Campgrounds

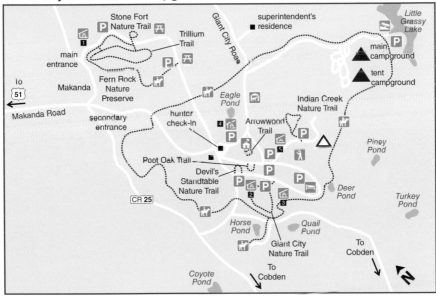

GETTING THERE

From the north, take I-57 to IL 13 West (Exit 54B). Drive west 13 miles to Giant City Road (there's a light, and a Walmart on the right). Turn left and go 12 miles south.

From the south, take I-57 to IL 148 West (Exit 45). Go 3 miles northwest to Grassy Road. Turn left. Go 9 miles to T-intersection with Giant City Road (stay left at fork at about 4.5 miles). Turn left and drive 4 miles to the park.

GPS COORDINATES: N37° 36.627'   W89° 10.984'

37

⛺ Hamilton County State Fish and Wildlife Area

Beauty ★★★★★ Privacy ★★★★ Spaciousness ★★★ Quiet ★★★★ Security ★★★★★ Cleanliness ★★★★★

Virtually every campsite at Hamilton County boasts an excellent view of the lake.

Over the years, the state of Illinois has taken advantage of its shallow valleys, rolling hills, and innumerable creeks to construct small recreational lakes that serve as the centerpiece of a number of parks and natural areas. I love these places—sometimes I enjoy fishing, but mostly I just love to hike and camp or even simply sit and relax near the open water.

Of all these, Hamilton County State Fish and Wildlife Area is certainly one of my favorites. The lake is beautiful, and the staff and campground hosts are friendly and helpful. You can fish or hike a few short trails, but most visitors come just to relax. Best of all, the campground is perfectly positioned on a wide point jutting into Dolan Lake and has been laid out so that virtually every site has an excellent view of the lake, which borders the campground on three sides. The tall trees throughout provide ample shade yet leave it feeling open and airy.

As you enter Hamilton County off IL 14, turn left and follow the signs south to the Piney Wood camping area. The main campground entrance will be on the left; just past it on the right is a small parking area, followed by four cabins. Park here to access the 10 walk-in sites, just to the west. These are great for tent campers—just enough of a walk to keep them underutilized but still readily accessible and close to the main campground's excellent facilities.

The rental cabins here feature a beautiful vista of Dolan Lake.

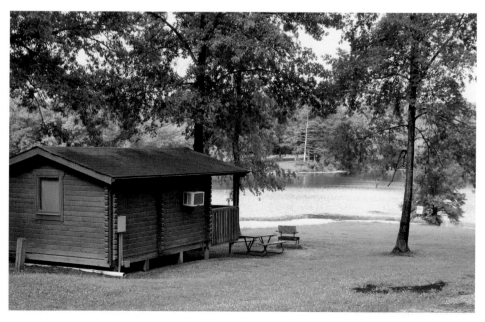

KEY INFORMATION

LOCATION: County Road 1625 E, McLeansboro, IL

CONTACT: 618-773-4340, bit.ly/HamiltonCtyIL

OPERATED BY: IDNR

OPEN: Year-round

SITES: Class A: 60 sites; Class C: 10 walk-in sites; 5 cabins

EACH SITE HAS: Picnic table, ground grill; electricity (Class A only)

WHEELCHAIR ACCESS: Restrooms and at least one accessible electric site

ASSIGNMENT: First come, first served; reservations available online (Class A and cabins only)

REGISTRATION: Register first with the campground host (if available), or set up, then park staff will come by.

AMENITIES: Water spigots, vault toilets, shower house

PARKING: At site (Class A); in lot (Class C)

FEE: Class A: $20/night, $30/night holidays; Class C: $8/night; cabin: $45/night; $5 reservation fee

ELEVATION: 459'

RESTRICTIONS:

PETS: On leash only

QUIET HOURS: 10 p.m.–7 a.m.

FIRES: In fire rings only

ALCOHOL: Permitted

VEHICLES: 2 per site

OTHER: 14-day limit; 1 camping unit (RV or tent) or 2 smaller tents per site; 4 adults or 1 family of 6 per site

Walk down a little dip and back up, and site 1 is on the left. If it isn't already taken, this is my first choice—spacious, airy, and well shaded, with a gorgeous view of the lake, and just 300 feet from the parking lot. A bit farther down the trail are sites 2 and 3, which face each other and thus are a bit too neighborly. Site 4 is off by itself, 450 feet from parking, and is comfortably situated under tall pine trees. Site 5 is in a clearing but is a bit too close to the trail, and sites 6 and 7 are a bit farther down and face each other. Sites 8, 9, and 10 are grouped together at the end of the trail, a hike of about 700 feet from your car. I would pick one of these only if the other two in the group were unoccupied—and the chances of that are pretty good on an average nonholiday weekend.

Once you've selected your site, go to site 22 in the main campground to register with the campground host. You can fill water containers at the spigot by the tent-camping parking lot and use the restrooms and showers at the large clean shower house just across the road in the main campground. The shower house was built in 1997 but is so well maintained that I first thought it was erected much more recently. It's heated and open year-round to all campers.

If you want electricity, or just like the convenience of being able to park at your campsite, the main campground also has some beautiful spots on the lake. As you drive into the campground, the first right is a short spur with sites 21–25, the shower house, a playground, and the campground host, from whom you can purchase ice, soft drinks, and fishing bait. Next is an intersection, where you'll find the toilet. Turn right for sites 1–20, or go straight or left for sites 26–57. This campground is much busier on the weekends, and you'll be sharing with RVs, but the lakeside sites are attractive and fairly large. Check out any of the sites 7–16, 34, 35, or 37.

Friends or family who can't handle too much roughing it can reserve (well in advance!) one of the five cabins. These are located next to the tent parking area and offer the same beautiful lakefront view, plus beds for six, a grill, a table and chairs, heat, air-conditioning, and fans. The cabins and all the Class A sites can be reserved online at reserveamerica.com for an additional $5.

Dolan Lake is the centerpiece of the area, with more than 3 miles of shoreline and a half-dozen serene picnic areas situated around it. You can sit and read a book, enjoy the view, or take a nap. For a little more exercise, stroll the trails that start from the campground and encircle most of the lake. Fishing is also excellent, since the lake was drained, refilled, and restocked a few years ago with largemouth bass, bluegill, catfish, and crappie.

The small Dolan Lake concession on the other side of the lake has unfortunately been closed for several years. You will find plenty of stores and restaurants, though, in nearby McLeansboro, just 8 miles west on IL 14.

Hamilton County State Fish and Wildlife Area: Piney Wood Campground

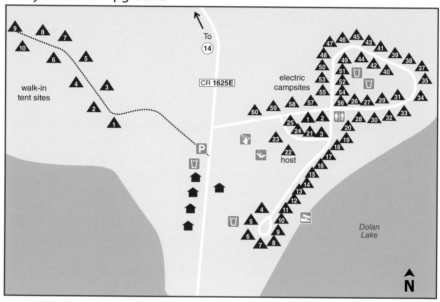

GETTING THERE

From McLeansboro, go 7 miles east on IL 14. Turn right onto CR 1625 East at the park sign. Go 1.1 miles south to the park entrance, on the right.

GPS COORDINATES: N38° 03.997'   W88° 24.266'

38

Lake Murphysboro State Park

Beauty ★★★★ Privacy ★★★ Spaciousness ★★★ Quiet ★★★★ Security ★★★★ Cleanliness ★★★★★

Half of the tent sites are as close to the lake as you can get without a boat.

I love camping at the water's edge, whether it be by a lake, creek, or rolling river. I love it even more when a park like Lake Murphysboro has taken advantage of its miles of shoreline to set up two completely separate lakeside camping areas, one primarily for RVs, and one for tents. And we tent campers get the better deal—our campground is smaller, quieter, and closer to the lake.

After you turn north off IL 149 into the park, turn right toward Lake Murphysboro. If you go straight into the park, you'll come to the popular Big Oak Campground, with 54 electric campsites. Turn left instead, and continue north around the lake 0.5 mile to the two adjacent tent-camping areas (20 sites total). Each site has a table, ground grill, and lantern pole, and most are located on the lakeshore—perfectly situated for fishing, or just sitting and enjoying the view. The first five sites, called Water Lily Campground, are between the main park road and the lake. Site 4 is designated wheelchair-accessible; there are vault toilets directly across the road. Though they're attractive, the primary disadvantage of these sites is their proximity to the road. For that reason, I prefer the sites just around the corner, along the dead-end Shady Rest Campground road.

There's plenty of access for boating and fishing along the shores of Lake Murphysboro.   *photo by Karas Hall*

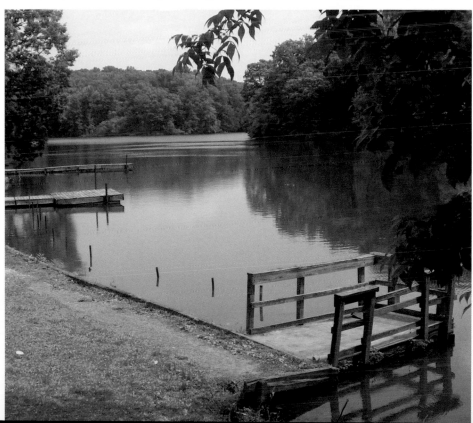

KEY INFORMATION

LOCATION: 52 Cinder Hill Drive, Murphysboro, IL 62966

CONTACT: 618-684-2867, bit.ly/LakeMurphysboroIL

OPERATED BY: IDNR

OPEN: Year-round

SITES: Class A: 54 electric; Class B: 20 nonelectric

EACH SITE HAS: Picnic table, fire ring or ground grill, lantern pole

WHEELCHAIR ACCESS: Restrooms and at least one accessible tent site

ASSIGNMENT: First come, first served; reservations available online

REGISTRATION: Set up and register with host in Big Oak Campground or park staff will come by

AMENITIES: Water spigots, vault toilets, shower house

PARKING: At site

FEE: Class A: $20/night, $30/night holidays; Class B: $10/night ($8 when showers closed); $5 reservation fee

ELEVATION: 494'

RESTRICTIONS:

PETS: On leash only

QUIET HOURS: 10 p.m.–7 a.m.

FIRES: In fire rings only

ALCOHOL: Permitted

VEHICLES: 2 per site

OTHER: 14-day limit; 1 RV and 1 tent, or 2 tents per site; 4 adults or 1 family per site

Shady Rest has 15 sites, half of them as close to the lake as you can get without a boat. Sites 1, 2, and 3 on the right as you enter are good—3 has more space and shade. Sites 4 and 8 are small, but site 5, which is between them, is attractive. All the other sites are spacious, but my favorite is site 15, at the end of the road, which has more room to spread out beneath some tree cover.

Once you've selected an unreserved site, register with the campground host at the first site in Big Oak Campground, or settle in and park staff will come by later. There are vault toilets at both campgrounds, but you'll need to get water at the shower house on the other side of the lake.

The tent areas don't fill up as often as the RV campground, but they're still about half full on most good weekends. You can reserve selected sites in advance via reserveamerica .com for an additional $5.

The main park road makes a loop around the lake, a scenic drive with several turnoffs leading to wooded picnic areas on lakeside promontories. On the opposite side of the lake from the campgrounds you'll find the boat launch and shower house, open to all campers from April 1–late December (depending on weather). Around the lake are numerous places to bank fish, as well as a beautiful wooden wheelchair-accessible fishing pier by the docks. There is no boat rental or concession, but you'll find plenty of stores and restaurants in nearby Murphysboro.

Considerably more open water and recreational opportunities can be found down the road at nearby Kinkaid Lake. Head straight west out of Lake Murphysboro along Lake Access Road, which becomes Marina Road and curves right at 1.4 miles. Another 1.4 miles brings you to the Kinkaid Village Marina, where you'll find a restaurant (open weekends), boat rental, groceries, ice, fishing tackle, and bait, as well as a very busy RV campground. The marina is open April–mid-October. You can reach them at 618-687-4914 for more information. This area is hopping on most summer weekends, with hordes of boaters, fishermen, water-skiers, and house-boaters. However, the lake offers 2,750 surface acres, more than 90 miles of shoreline, and almost 9,300 acres of surrounding wilderness, so there are plenty of places to get away from the crowds by boat, foot, or mountain bike.

The lands south and west of Kinkaid Lake are part of the Shawnee National Forest and feature more than 30 miles of fairly rugged trails, with several trailheads and possible routes between them. One beautiful hike begins at the dam at the southern end of the lake and winds north along the lakeshore 3 miles to the Buttermilk Hill picnic area. When you reach the forest service road at the end of the point, turn right to go down to the picnic area and restrooms. (You'll have to retrace your steps to the dam, since the picnic area is accessible by boat or foot only.) To get to the dam, go west on IL 149 to Spillway Road (just past the bridge). Turn right and head north 1.25 miles to the parking area in front of the gate. The trail begins 0.25 mile up the hill, at the west end of the dam. For a map and descriptions of this and other trails in the area, go to bit.ly/KinkaidLakeTrailMap. As on all trails in the Shawnee Forest, be sure to carry water, a map, and a compass or GPS unit.

Lake Murphysboro State Park: Water Lily and Shady Rest Campgrounds

GETTING THERE

From US 51 and IL 13 in Carbondale, go west 7 miles to Murphysboro, where IL 13 becomes IL 149. Continue 3.5 miles west on IL 149 to Lake Access Road, on the right. Turn right and go 0.5 mile to the park entrance, also on the right.

GPS COORDINATES: N37° 46.639'   W89° 23.327'

39

⛺ Pere Marquette State Park

Beauty ★★★★★ Privacy ★★★ Spaciousness ★★★★ Quiet ★★★★ Security ★★★★★ Cleanliness ★★★★★

The climb to McAdams Peak is a workout, but the view of the Illinois River below is ample reward.

I have long loved hiking the trails at Pere Marquette, with their bluffs and stunning views. I didn't include it in the first edition of this book, however, because I assumed the campground was always crowded. And the 78-site RV section usually is. Then one beautiful summer weekend I decided to try out the tent area—and I was converted. Of the 20 or so sites available, most are spread out and spacious, and only 2 others were occupied that weekend. Add to that the beautiful lodge and restaurant that's a short walk from the campground, and Pere Marquette is now in the book.

Appropriately, you start your visit to Pere Marquette at the visitor center, just to the left as you enter the park off IL 100. The center has a 3-D map of the area as well as some fascinating natural history displays. (Let the kids climb inside the life-size replica of an eagle's nest.) Here you can register for a campsite and pick up trail maps and other area information. (You can also register with the host in the RV campground.)

The main campground entrance is 0.5 mile east of the visitor center on IL 100. Drive past the RV area and shower house (which all campers can use) to the tent-camping area on the north side. Here you'll find about 21 unnumbered sites scattered around a large loop, determined mostly by wherever you find a table and fire grate. You can park on the

Overlook at McAdams Peak, along the Ridge Trail

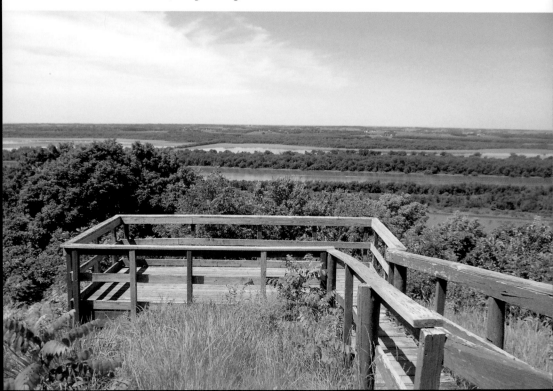

KEY INFORMATION

LOCATION: 13112 Visitor Center Lane, Grafton IL 62037

CONTACT: 618-786-3323, bit.ly/PereMarquetteIL

OPERATED BY: IDNR

OPEN: Year-round

SITES: Class A: 78 sites; Class B: 21 sites; 2 cabins

EACH SITE HAS: Picnic table, ground grill; electricity at Class A only

WHEELCHAIR ACCESS: Restrooms and at least one accessible electric site

ASSIGNMENT: First come, first served; reservations available online (Class A & cabins only)

REGISTRATION: Register at the visitor center or with the campground host

AMENITIES: Water spigots, vault toilets, shower house

PARKING: At site or nearby

FEE: Class A: $20/night, $30/night holidays; Class B: $10/night; Cabin: $45/night; $5 reservation fee

ELEVATION: 525'

RESTRICTIONS:

PETS: On leash only

FIRES: In fire rings only

ALCOHOL: Permitted

VEHICLES: 2 per site

OTHER: 14-day limit; 1 RV and 1 tent, or 2 tents per site; 4 adults or 1 family per site

---

grass near most sites. If you want plenty of space and a bit more isolation, sites 8–11 off the northeast corner (numbered on my map for reference) are a good choice. My favorites are a short walk from the small parking areas on the north side of the loop. Sites 12 and 13 are north of the road, beautifully shaded and secluded. Sites 15 and 16 are all by themselves, perched atop the hill in the middle of the loop.

The tent area is not nearly as popular as the RV section, but you will find it busy on some weekends, particularly in October, when fall foliage draws more campers. If you want more solitude, camp midweek during the busy seasons, or camp at McCully Heritage Project, 25 miles north on IL 100.

For any companions who want a bit (or a lot) more luxury, Pere Marquette offers plenty of choices. In addition to the RV sites with electric hookups, the campground has two simple camping cabins, with beds, electricity, heat, and air (but no indoor cooking or plumbing). The RV sites and cabins can be reserved online through reserveamerica.com. For more comfort, check out the rooms and stone cottages at the Pere Marquette Lodge. Call 618-786-2331 or check pmlodge.net for information and reservations.

Even if your preferences (or budget) preclude you from staying there, the beautiful lodge is well worth visiting. Grab a comfortable chair in the lobby, admire its massive timbers and huge 700-ton stone fireplace, and read or just look out over the Illinois River. Use the money you've saved by tent camping to splurge on a great meal at the restaurant. Note that the lodge hosts a variety of special events throughout the year—click the events tab on their website to see what might be coming up.

I've hiked all 12 miles of trail at Pere Marquette, and one of my favorites is a 2-mile combination of the Dogwood, Ridge, and Goat Cliff Trails. Pick up the Dogwood Trail just north of the visitor center, climb up (and up) to the Ridge Trail and on to the overlook at McAdams Peak. It's a workout to get there, but the breathtaking view of the Illinois River below is ample reward. Continue north on Goat Cliff to more overlooks, then descend alongside the bluffs back to the visitor center. Pick up the color-coded trail map there to explore the rest—they're all well maintained and signed.

There's no lack of other things to do in and around Pere Marquette. You can rent a bike at the lodge and pedal the paved 20-mile Sam Vadalabene Trail along the Illinois and Mississippi Rivers, or explore the rivers on a guided boat tour (graftonharbor.net). The Pere Marquette Stables offer guided horseback trail rides and hayrides (graftontrailrides.com). Venture into nearby Grafton for shops, restaurants, a zipline (aeriesview.com), and a water park (ragingrivers.com). You'll sleep well back in your tent at night!

Pere Marquette State Park: Tent Campground

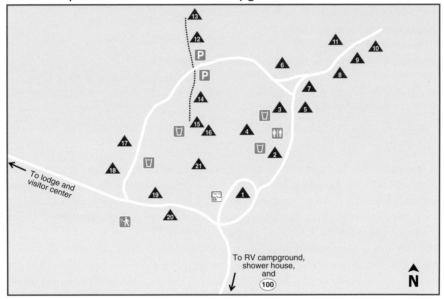

GETTING THERE

From Alton, take IL 100 west 21 miles to the park entrance on the right.

GPS COORDINATES: N42° 21.518'   W89° 19.277'

40

Pine Hills Campground

Beauty ★★★★ Privacy ★★★ Spaciousness ★★★ Quiet ★★★★★ Security ★★★★ Cleanliness ★★★★★

Prepare to be awed by the impressive bluffs of the LaRue–Pine Hills.

Geologically, southwestern Illinois around the Pine Hills is much more like Missouri than Illinois. These narrow ridges and steep hillsides are more reminiscent of the Ozarks to the west and, in fact, represent the easternmost edge of what geologists call the Ozark Uplift. Fortunately for Illinois, the Mississippi River intervened and carved this area from the plateau by its millennia-long wanderings. The result is a virtual island of spectacular bluffs and amazing biodiversity.

In the midst of this, Pine Hills Campground is a simple, quiet retreat. With few amenities and only 13 campsites, it doesn't attract RVs, and it is a perfect base camp for exploring the more than 21,000 acres of eastern Shawnee Forest wilderness that surround it.

The campground consists of a single 0.25-mile road, along which the campsites sit. There is no water, but there are vault toilets between sites 10 and 11. Each site has a table, a fire ring, and a lantern post. As you enter the campground, you'll see the signboard and self-registration post on the right. Once you've selected your site, come back here to register and deposit your fee.

Looking up at the bluffs at LaRue–Pine Hills

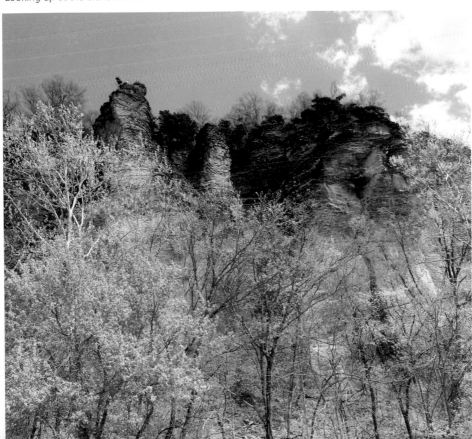

KEY INFORMATION

LOCATION: Pine Hills Road, Wolf Lake, IL 62998

CONTACT: Mississippi Bluffs Ranger District, 618-833-8576, bit.ly/PineHillsIL

OPERATED BY: U.S. Forest Service

OPEN: March 15–December 15

SITES: 13 tent sites

EACH SITE HAS: Picnic table, fire ring, lantern pole

WHEELCHAIR ACCESS: Restrooms and at least one accessible tent site

ASSIGNMENT: First come, first served

REGISTRATION: Register at the self-registration post at the entrance

AMENITIES: Vault toilets

PARKING: At site

FEE: $10/night

ELEVATION: 415'

RESTRICTIONS:

PETS: On leash only

QUIET HOURS: 10 p.m.–6 a.m.

FIRES: In fire rings only

ALCOHOL: Permitted

VEHICLES: 2 per site

OTHER: 14-day limit; 8 campers per site

Sites 1–8 are immediately visible in the first section of the campground, in a grassy clearing with some shade, surrounded by woods. Although sufficiently spacious and spread out, they don't offer much of a sense of privacy. I suggest heading back to sites 9–13, which are more separated from the rest of the campground. These offer much better shade and more seclusion. Site 13, at the end of the loop, is my favorite, tucked back into the surrounding woods a bit.

While at Pine Hills, don't miss the nearby LaRue–Pine Hills Research Natural Area. Here the limestone bluffs of the Ozark Plateaus face west, overlooking the swamps at their base. You can get there by heading north from the campground on Pine Hills Road, but to appreciate the bluffs you should approach from the west. Take Pine Hills Road south to State Forest Road, then head right to reach IL 3. Turn right again, continue 4.6 miles, and make another right, onto Muddy Levee Road, just before the bridge over Big Muddy River. Follow the Big Muddy for about 2 miles, and then, when you curve to the right, away from the river, the bluffs jump into view. Another 0.5 mile takes you to the base of the bluffs and the intersection with LaRue Road.

From the road below, you might barely see little people looking down from several hundred feet above you. To get to where they are, turn left at the T-intersection, go 0.3 mile, and turn right, onto Pine Hills Road. Go 0.7 mile uphill, to the parking area on the right labeled "Inspiration Point." A 0.25-mile hike will reward you with a panoramic view of the Mississippi River valley below. If you look carefully, you should be able to discern in the swamp the rounded edges of the Mississippi's erstwhile channel. Don't stop there, though. Continue another 500 feet to a couple of other excellent vistas. If you're surefooted and choose to ignore the signs telling you to stay on the trail, there are some obviously worn paths leading out to the bluff's edge.

If you're not herpetophobic, twice a year you can experience another natural wonder at LaRue–Pine Hills, this one biological: the biannual snake migration. The swamp is home to more than half the reptile and amphibian species found in Illinois, including 35 types of snakes. Each fall, with the drop in temperature, they all migrate from the swamp, across LaRue Road to hibernate in the bluffs—then they head back in the spring. A 2.5-mile segment of the road is closed from March 15–May 15, and from September 1–October 30 to allow them to cross. You can park at the lot by Winters Pond, just to the right (south) of the junction of Big Muddy Levee Road and LaRue Road, and hike from there. You won't see masses of snakes. When I hiked it one pleasant April morning, I encountered two cottonmouths, two timber rattlers, and one little green snake, all quietly basking in the sun.

Hikers can explore many miles of rugged trails in the area, starting with White Pine Trail, which begins just behind campsite 10. The trail comes to a junction at about 0.8 mile—continuing straight ahead another 1.2 miles takes you to the clear waters of Hutchins Creek, while heading left takes you along the ridgeline another 2.2 miles to Allen's Flat picnic area on Pine Hills Road. A basic trail map can be found at bit.ly/WhitePineTrailIL. If you're more ambitious, try the 6-mile Godwin Trail, which crosses the Clear Springs and Bald Knob Wilderness areas. The western trailhead is on Pine Hills Road, about 5.7 miles north of the campground. A trail description can be found at bit.ly/GodwinBackpackerIL. For this and other wilderness trails, a topographic map and compass or GPS unit are highly recommended.

Pine Hills Campground

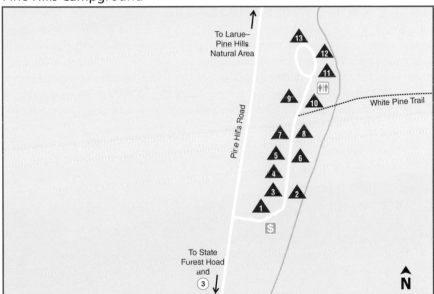

GETTING THERE

From Jonesboro, take IL 146 west to IL 3. Turn right, go 4.25 miles north to State Forest Road. Turn right again and go 0.6 mile east to Pine Hills Road. Turn left and drive 0.7 mile north to the campground entrance, on the right.

From Murphysboro, take IL 127 south 21 miles to State Forest Road. Turn right and go 7 miles west to Pine Hills Road. Turn right again and proceed as above.

GPS COORDINATES: N37° 30.870'   W89° 25.384'

41

Pounds Hollow Recreation Area:
PINE RIDGE CAMPGROUND

Beauty ★★★★ Privacy ★★★★ Spaciousness ★★ Quiet ★★★★★ Security ★★★★ Cleanliness ★★★★

Pine Ridge is an underappreciated gem, where you can camp in a beautiful pine wood near a tranquil beach.

Pine Ridge Campground in the Pounds Hollow Recreation Area has to be one of the most underappreciated camping gems in southern Illinois. While it once had 75 sites, half of these are closed most of the time, with some opened as overflow during exceptionally busy times. Since Pine Ridge has limited facilities and no shower, it's not popular with the RV crowd. A fair-weather nonholiday weekend may only see 5–10 sites occupied—which is all the better for those of us who don't mind tent camping in a beautiful pine wood, near a tranquil beach, great hiking, and all the attractions of the eastern Shawnee National Forest.

As you enter the recreation area, take the left fork to go to the campground. Pass the two closed camping loops, containing sites 1–13, and 14–35. You'll come to the first open camping spur off to the left, with sites 54–76, and then a little farther on, the spur with sites 36–53.

As the name suggests, all the sites are nicely shaded under stately, tall pines. Each has a table, a ground grill, and a lantern pole, and sufficient room for a tent or two. They aren't far apart, but since the campground is rarely busy, you should find plenty of privacy. I prefer the spur containing sites 36–53, where the sites are more spacious. As a bonus, all but site 42 here have an electric hookup, and unlike most places there is no extra charge. Sites 46, 47,

The scenic beach at Pounds Hollow Lake

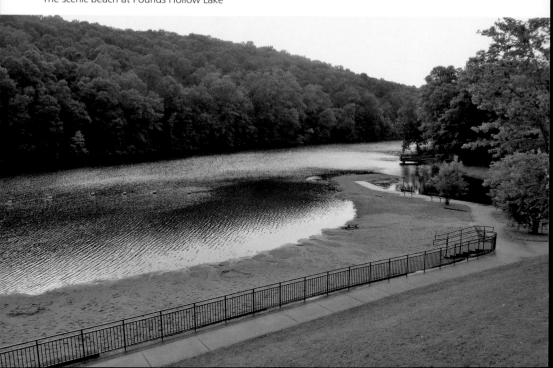

KEY INFORMATION

LOCATION: Pounds Hollow Road, Junction, IL 62954

CONTACT: Hidden Springs Ranger District, 618-658-2111, bit.ly/PineRidgeIL

OPERATED BY: U.S. Forest Service

OPEN: March 1–December 15

SITES: 39

EACH SITE HAS: Picnic table, fire ring, and lantern pole; electricity (13 sites)

WHEELCHAIR ACCESS: Restrooms and at least one accessible tent site

ASSIGNMENT: First come, first served

REGISTRATION: Register at the self-registration post at the entrance

AMENITIES: Water spigot, vault toilets

PARKING: At site

FEE: $10/night

ELEVATION: 651'

RESTRICTIONS:

PETS: On leash only

QUIET HOURS: 10 p.m.–6 a.m.

FIRES: In fire rings only

ALCOHOL: Permitted

VEHICLES: 2 per site

OTHER: 14-day limit; 8 campers per site

and 48, toward the end of the spur, are good choices. In the other section, I like 56, 61, 73, and 75 for shade and space. Unlike at some campgrounds, the sites in the loops at the end of the road are smaller and not as good. There are vault toilets in both spurs, but the only water spigot is at the campground entrance, across from the information board.

Once you've selected your site, as with most campgrounds in the Shawnee National Forest, return to the campground entrance to register and pay at the self-registration post.

Back at the recreation-area entrance, take the right fork, and you'll be on the one-way loop headed to Pounds Hollow Lake and a very picturesque and quiet beach. The Civilian Conservation Corps constructed the beach area in 1938, and their excellent work can still be seen in the hand-cut sandstone foundation of the picnic shelter. It has recently been refurbished, and now has a beautiful picnic area, changing rooms, flush toilets, a cold-water "shower tower" on the beach, and some nice fishing areas off to the north side. It's not a big beach, but it's usually not crowded—and it's free!

I enjoy a day of warming up with hiking in the morning and cooling off with swimming in the afternoon, and Pounds Hollow makes that easy. At the end of the beach is part of Beaver Trail, which leads to the canyons, shelter caves, and an overlook of Rim Rock Recreation Trail. You'll reach Rim Rock in just 0.5 mile and can explore the cool canyons below. Be sure to check out Ox-Lot Cave, a historic shelter bluff cave. Climb the stairway to the 0.8-mile loop trail above, where you'll see the remnants of an American Indian wall, and look out over Pounds Hollow Lake. Near the stairwell is "Fat Man's Misery," where you can squeeze through huge boulders. The trail is well marked and designated "hiker-only" for this portion, so you won't be sharing it with horses. Water and toilets are available at the Rim Rock parking area, off the loop trail above.

You can also hike Beaver Trail in the other direction, starting from the earthen dam at the north end of the lake. The trail runs a total of 9 miles to Camp Cadiz, but the most interesting portion is the first mile, to Karbers Ridge Road; you'll go up and down hills, past creeks, and by rocky outcrops.

If Pine Ridge suits you as a base camp, you can, in fact, explore much of the eastern Shawnee Forest from there. Pounds Hollow is conveniently close to the must-see Garden of the Gods. From the park entrance, go 6.6 miles west on Karbers Ridge Road, then head 1.4 miles north. (See the Pharaoh Campground profile on page 134 for more details.) Even closer, though, is the less famous High Knob, a 929-foot sandstone prominence with a 2-mile loop trail and some excellent views. Travel 5 miles west of Pounds Hollow on Karbers Ridge Road, then 1.6 miles north on CR 2 to Knob Hill. Make a right about 0.8 mile up the hill and pass the horse camp to reach the High Knob picnic area.

Pounds Hollow Recreation Area: Pine Ridge Campground

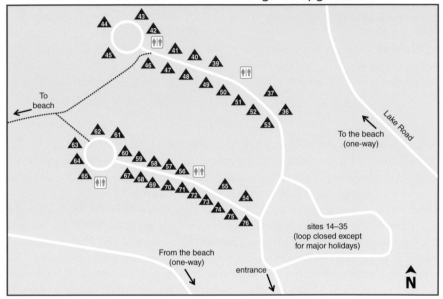

GETTING THERE

From Harrisburg, take IL 34 south 15.3 miles to Karbers Ridge Road. Turn left and go 9.5 miles (this becomes Pounds Hollow Road at about 8 miles) to the Pounds Hollow sign. Turn left.

From IL 1, turn west onto CR 13/Pounds Hollow Road. Drive 1.9 miles to the Pounds Hollow sign and turn right.

GPS COORDINATES: N37° 36.725'   W88° 16.038'

42

Pyramid State Recreation Area

Beauty ★★★ Privacy ★★★★★ Spaciousness ★★★ Quiet ★★★★★ Security ★★★★ Cleanliness ★★★★★

Come find your own private lake for camping, fishing, and even canoeing.

If you like to camp in places not quite so tame, Pyramid State Recreation Area might be for you. With more than 19,000 acres, Pyramid is Illinois's largest state park, almost all of it on land that was once strip-mined for coal. Time and man's intervention have restored the land to a haven for wildlife, a rugged mix of heavily forested hills, meadows, wetlands, and dozens of small lakes. Hunters, fishermen, hikers, and campers can all find plenty of room to get away.

Most visitors will spend their time in what's called the "Original Pyramid," the 3,200 acres first designated as a state park in 1968. That's where you'll find the park office and three primitive campgrounds with 48 total sites, plus about 11 hike-in campsites. All sites have a picnic table and ground grill, and each campground has vault toilets. The only water spigot is located at the park office, by the entrance. Most of the vehicular access sites are small, though there are some lakeside gems among them. Outside of archery season (October 1–mid-January), Pyramid sees very few campers—and even then, less than a quarter of sites will be occupied on the busiest weekend.

One of the many little lakes that dot the landscape at Pyramid State Recreation Area   *photo by Karas Hall*

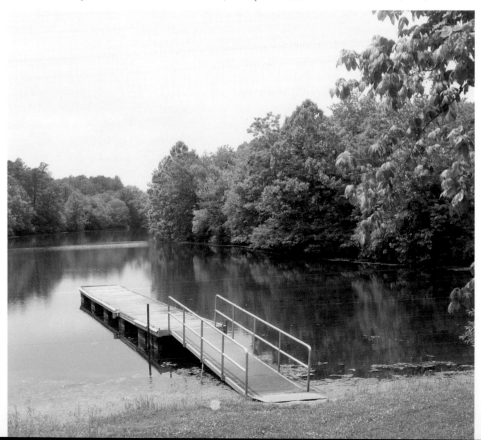

KEY INFORMATION

LOCATION: 1562 Pyramid Park Road, Pinckneyville, IL

CONTACT: 618-357-2574, bit.ly/PyramidIL

OPERATED BY: IDNR

OPEN: Year-round

SITES: Class C: 48 sites; Class D: 11 hike-in sites

EACH SITE HAS: Table, ground grill

WHEELCHAIR ACCESS: Not designated

ASSIGNMENT: First come, first served

REGISTRATION: Register at the office or at the self-registration post if the office is closed

AMENITIES: Water spigot (at office only), vault toilets

PARKING: At campsite; at nearest parking lot for hike-in sites

FEE: Class C: $8 per tent; hike-in sites: $6/night

ELEVATION: 410'

RESTRICTIONS:

PETS: On leash only

QUIET HOURS: 10 p.m.–7 a.m.

FIRES: In fire rings only

ALCOHOL: Permitted

VEHICLES: 2 per site

OTHER: 14-day limit; 2 tents or 1 RV per site; 4 adults or 1 family per site

As you enter Pyramid, take the first left at the office (where you'll return to register, either with staff or at the self-registration post) and go straight back to Heron Campground. Heron has nine sites laid out in a row along the north side of the road, with a fence and croplands to the south. These sites are flat and grassy, with woods behind and trees around, providing plenty of shade. Though not widely separated, these are the largest pull-in campsites at Pyramid. I like site 2 because it's set back from the road a bit. Pyramid doesn't draw many RVs because there's no electricity or water hookups, but Heron is the one campground where you may occasionally see a small pop-up or trailer.

To get to Boulder Lake Campground, turn left out of Heron, go north, and turn right at the T-intersection. The road ends at the campground, with sites 1–9 to the left and 10–18 to the right. Site 1, at the north end, is right on Boulder Lake and next to the boat ramp, and site 11 offers the most space and a bit of seclusion, with some surrounding brush and trees. Sites 2–10, 17, and 18 are tiny and too close together. The small field and grove of trees past site 14 at the south end contains eight sites for equestrians only.

The North Campground at Pyramid is on the opposite side of the park. From the entrance, go straight past the office and follow the road all the way to the northeast corner, where the campground with 19 sites is tucked between five small lakes. The better sites are located at either end of the campground road, next to the lakes. To the right (east), sites 21, 22, and 23 are small, but in a very pretty spot by themselves on Clear Lake. If no one else is camping nearby, 23 in particular is a good choice. At the west end (to the left), sites 4, 5, and 7–11 are good, situated between Beehive and Plum Lakes. Site 5 is perched atop a small hill by itself, and site 7 is my favorite; it's fairly large, right on Beehive Lake, and near a small fishing dock. (Sites 1, 2, 3, and 6 no longer exist.) The sites in the middle are too small and close together.

If you want real seclusion and don't mind walking a bit, Pyramid has 11 separate hike-in sites, ranging from 200 yards to 1 mile from the nearest parking lot. Several are right on the water, so with a little effort you can have your own private lake for camping, fishing, and canoeing. There is a beautiful site on Hook Lake, about 0.5 mile from the nearest lot. To get there, go north past the office and the archery range to the parking area on the curve. From there take the trail heading downhill to the west. You'll find one site along the trail at about 0.4 mile, but continue another 500 feet to the one on the lake. Most of the hike-in sites have a table, ground grill, and trashcan. Note that not all the hike-in sites on older park maps are currently maintained. Check in at the office before camping, both to register and to find out which sites are usable and where to park for easiest access.

The 16.5 miles of trails at Pyramid are wide and well maintained and are open to hikers, equestrians, and even mountain bikers. Pyramid attracts plenty of wildlife, and you're likely to see deer, wild turkey, migrating waterfowl (in season)—and ticks. When I was there in the spring, ticks weren't noticeable at the campgrounds, but I picked up quite a collection while hiking the trails. Take the necessary precautions (see page 7), or plan to camp in the fall when they're not as prevalent.

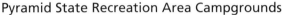

Pyramid State Recreation Area Campgrounds

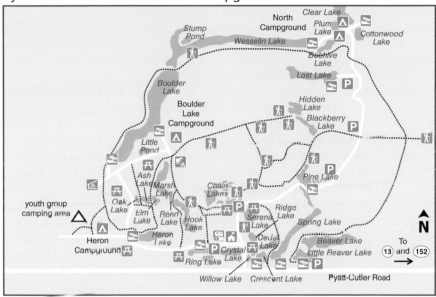

GETTING THERE

From US 51 in DuQuoin, head 9.6 miles west on IL 152 (Main Street, which becomes Pyatt-Cutler Road at 6.8 miles) to the park entrance, on the right.

From the junction of IL 154 and IL 13 in Pinckneyville (Main and Water Streets), go 5.5 miles south on IL 13 to Pyatt Cutler Road. Turn right and drive 2.5 miles to the park entrance on the right.

GPS COORDINATES: N38° 00.269'   W89° 24.989'

43

⛺ Randolph County State Recreation Area

Beauty ★★★ Privacy ★★★ Spaciousness ★★★ Quiet ★★★★ Security ★★★★ Cleanliness ★★★★★

This underappreciated camping getaway is neither too busy nor too far from some unique natural venues.

Randolph County State Recreation Area is another of the underappreciated camping getaways in southern Illinois; it's neither too busy nor too far from some interesting natural venues. Among the three campgrounds, the one with electric hookups draws most of the traffic, leaving the other two, which are less popular, available for tent campers.

Enter the park, arrive at a T-intersection, and turn right. The next left brings you into Oak Ridge, the smallest and least-used of Randolph County's three campgrounds. There are supposed to be 15 unnumbered sites here, but gauging from the ground grills and tables, I'd say there are 12 (numbered on my map for reference). Regardless, you can set up near any grill and move tables around as needed. Just park on the grass near your site. All these are good choices—site 9 is great for shade.

For a more scenic option, check out the two walk-in sites down by the lake. You can park in the loop past sites 11 and 12 to unload, and carry your gear down the steps to the lakefront, which is about 200 feet away. These are set apart from the other sites (up the hill), but be aware that those campers may come down to fish.

Down the road from the Oak Ridge entrance is the park office, where you register, and the Pine Ridge RV Campground—it has been recently renovated, but pass it up for tent camping. Head back north on the main park road, go past the road to the group campground, and take the next left to Rolling Hills Campground. Again, these sites are unnumbered; there are supposed to be 31, but I count 25. The sites are spread along the road and in two small loops to the north, each with a parking lot (though you can pull right up to

The view from the top of Fults Hill Prairie is worth the climb.

photo by David Walker

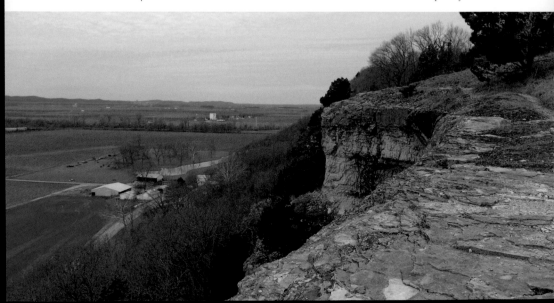

KEY INFORMATION

LOCATION: 4301 South Lake Drive, Chester, IL 62233

CONTACT: 618-826-2706, bit.ly/RandolphCtyIL

OPERATED BY: IDNR

OPEN: Year-round

SITES: Class B: 51 electric sites; Class C: 37 vehicle-access sites; Class D: 5 walk-in sites

EACH SITE HAS: Picnic table, ground grill; electricity (Class B only)

WHEELCHAIR ACCESS: Restrooms and at least one accessible tent site

ASSIGNMENT: First come, first served

REGISTRATION: Register at the park office

AMENITIES: Water spigots, vault toilets

PARKING: At site (Class B & C); in lot (Class D)

FEE: Class B: $18/night; Class C: $8/night; Class D: $6/night

ELEVATION: 510'

RESTRICTIONS:

PETS: On leash only

QUIET HOURS: 10 p.m.–7 a.m.

FIRES: In fire rings only

ALCOHOL: Permitted

VEHICLES: 2 per site

OTHER: 14-day limit; 1 RV and 1 tent, or 2 tents per site; 6 people per site

---

each site). The sites on the first loop, 1–6 on my map, have poor shade. Those at the far end of the second loop, sites 11–13, are more spacious and shaded. My other favorite is the last drive-in site, number 25.

If the campground is busy and you'd like a little more space, the walk-in sites at the end of the Rolling Hills road are a good choice. The first is conveniently close to the parking area and is well shaded. I prefer the second, about 100 feet down the trail. The third is another 170 feet and not worth the additional steps.

Fishing is popular here, and the clear lake is stocked with channel catfish, redear, bluegill, walleye, saugeye, and rainbow trout. While some sources mention a concession, it hasn't operated for several years, but you can head to nearby Chester for stores and restaurants. While you're there, check out the granite statues of characters from the comic strip *Popeye*, whose creator was born in Chester (chesterill.com/character-trail).

Just a few miles (as the crow flies) southwest of Randolph County is Piney Creek Ravine State Natural Area, a fascinating hiking destination, which contains the largest body of prehistoric rock art in Illinois. A fairly rugged 2.5-mile loop, the hike is nicest in the spring, when the creek and waterfalls are flowing.

From the park, go west 1 mile to Palestine Road, then make a left and drive 3.8 miles south to Van Zant Street in Chester, then take a left and make a right onto SR 3. Turn left (south) and go 11.5 miles to Hog Hill Road, where you'll see a brown Piney Creek sign. Turn left, drive 3.8 miles to a T-intersection, then make a right; the next left will put you on Rock Crusher Road. Go 1 mile to Piney Creek Road, then take a left and travel 1.6 miles to the parking area, on the left. Pick up the trail to the left of the parking area, between two fencerows. Hike a short distance to the grassy area on the right, and cross to the preserve entrance. Be careful as you cross the slippery wet sandstone streambed.

For a hiking workout that leads to some stunning views, head to the Fults Hill Prairie Nature Preserve, about 30 miles northwest of the Randolph County State Recreation Area. To most people, prairies are flat grasslands, but Fults Hill is a prairie growing on a steep bluff overlooking the Mississippi. To get there, take IL 3 north about 13.5 miles to Ruma. Turn left onto IL 155, go 6.7 miles to Bluff Road, then turn right. Proceed 6.9 miles to the parking area on the right. You can take the loop trail in either direction, but I suggest going counterclockwise, starting on the right. You'll first have to tackle the 200 steps up, but that makes the end of the hike easier and saves the best views for last. The total length is about 1.6 miles, counting several side spurs to overlooks.

Randolph County State Recreation Area

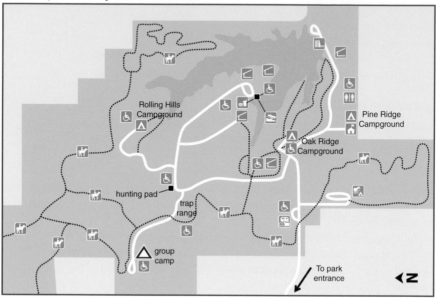

Randolph County State Recreation Area: Oak Ridge Campground

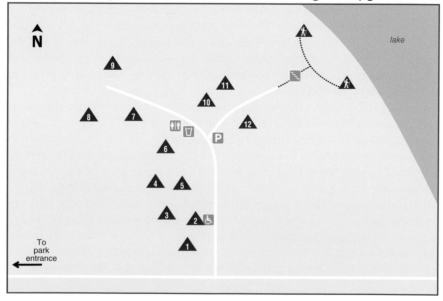

Randolph County State Recreation Area: Rolling Hills Campground

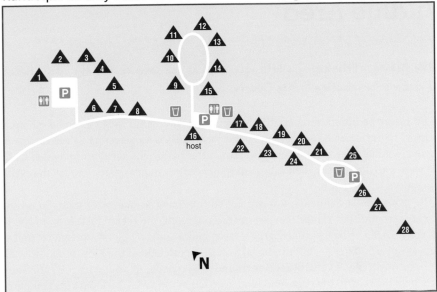

GETTING THERE

From the north, take IL 3 south 2.5 miles past Ellis Grove, to Shawneetown Trail. Turn left, go 3.6 miles east to Palestine Road. Turn right, go 1.6 miles, then make a left at the park entrance.

From the south, take IL 3 north to Chester. Turn right on State Street, go 0.3 mile to Van Zant Street, turn left, drive 0.25 mile to Palestine Road, and turn right. Travel 3.8 miles, then make a right at the park entrance.

GPS COORDINATES: N37° 58.317'   W89° 48.318'

44

Saline County State Fish and Wildlife Area

Beauty ★★★ Privacy ★★★ Spaciousness ★★★ Quiet ★★★ Security ★★★★★ Cleanliness ★★★★

A little fishing, a little hiking, a little relaxation as you camp next to the lake—these are good reasons for selecting Saline County.

A little fishing, a little hiking, a little relaxation as you camp next to the lakeshore, plus proximity to the Shawnee Forest—these are good reasons for selecting Saline County State Fish and Wildlife Area for a camping getaway. The 1,200-plus acres around Glen O. Jones Lake were once known for their salt springs (hence the county's name); today they serve as a recreational destination.

The campsites at Saline County are not concentrated in one place that you could call "the campground" but rather they are spread out along the rectangular loop of the main park road. Each site has a ground grill, a table, and a lantern pole; water spigots and vault toilets are nearby. Sites 1–23 face the lake on the south side of the loop, while sites 25–43 are on the north side, in grassy fields surrounded by woods. As you enter the park from the south, pass the road to the park office and head left at the fork. You'll pass the campground

Hike to the rugged sandstone bluff of Stone Face.

photo courtesy of Robert Pahre Photography

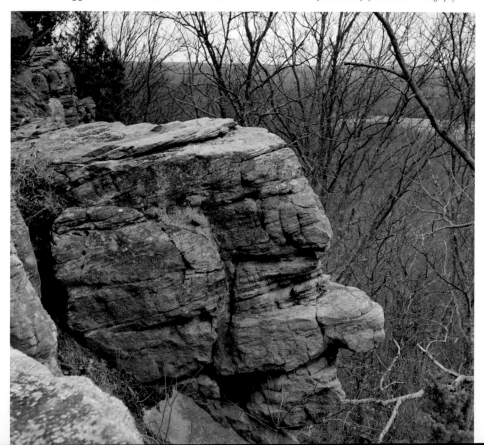

LOCATION: 85 Glen O. Jones Road, Equality, IL 62934

CONTACT: 618-276-4405, bit.ly/SalineCountyIL

OPERATED BY: IDNR

OPEN: Year-round

SITES: Class C: 43 sites

EACH SITE HAS: Picnic tables, fire pit and grill, lantern post

WHEELCHAIR ACCESS: Restrooms

ASSIGNMENT: First come, first served

REGISTRATION: Register with the campground host (if available) or set up and park staff will come by

AMENITIES: Water spigots, vault toilets

PARKING: At site

FEE: $8/night

ELEVATION: 381'

RESTRICTIONS:

PETS: On leash only

QUIET HOURS: 10 p.m.–7 a.m.

FIRES: In fire rings only

ALCOHOL: Permitted

VEHICLES: 2 per site

OTHER: 14-day limit; 1 RV and 1 tent, or 2 tents per site; 2 families per site

host, where you can register after you've selected your site. Sites 1–12 are the first you come to along the lakeshore. These are smaller, closer together, and popular but certainly offer a beautiful view of the lake. If you want one of these, site 4 would be my choice for space.

Sites 13 and 14 are on the southwest corner of the loop, and to the left is a parking lot for sites 15–23. These are also on the lake, and also popular, but if you want to fish or camp near water, this is the place to be. Site 19 is a bit bigger and is next to a floating dock good for fishing, but by far the best lakefront site is 23—flat, shaded, spacious, and all by itself on a point extending into the lake.

Up the hill and to the right are sites 25–43. Here you can spread out a bit more than down by the lake—sites are fairly spacious and level. They are grouped in sections along the road: sites 25–32 are together, then 33–35, then 36–39. Since these are not as popular as the lakefront sites, select a site in one of the latter two sections and you may end up with no campers nearby. The last four sites, 40–43, occupy a secluded wooded loop in the northeast corner of the park. This is labeled the equestrian area but isn't limited to campers with horses. However, park staff will tell you it's informally known as "the party area"—this is where groups that want to stay up later and be a little louder come to camp. If that's not you, this is probably an area to avoid on the weekends. During midweek or off-season, though, it should be a perfect place for privacy. Camping normally fills up only on holiday weekends—on any other fair-weather weekend, about half to two-thirds of the sites will be occupied.

Fishing is good at Saline County. You can bank or boat fish on 105-acre Glen O. Jones Lake for largemouth bass, bluegill, redear, crappie, and channel catfish. There are two launching ramps and two docks. You can also go after rainbow trout on the two-acre trout pond, which is stocked annually.

For hiking, there are four trails in the park. Lake Trail is 3 miles long, traveling around the lake from the dam to site 13. River Trail is 1 mile long, heading from the equestrian campground through woods down to the Saline River. Wildlife Nature Trail is a short, easy 0.75-mile loop in the middle of the park. Cave Hill Trail begins in the northwest corner of the park loop, by the bronze statue of Tecumseh. This is a more rugged 3-mile trail that ascends along a ridge with ravines on either side and climbs to Cave Hill, offering some excellent views of the surrounding countryside. It also leads to Equality Cave. However, the cave itself is gated by the U.S. Forest Service and is closed. It may reopen at some point, but if you're looking for a first "wild cave" to explore, Equality isn't a good choice. Even locals have gotten lost in this maze of a cave.

Just 6 miles from Saline County is another of the Shawnee National Forest's many interesting sandstone formations: Stone Face, which resembles, as you might expect, the side profile of a man's head. The moderately rugged loop trail to Stone Face is about 1.75 miles long and leads past a shelter cave and some impressive bluff views. From the Saline County park exit, turn left, go 0.5 mile north to CR 17 (Horseshoe Road), and turn left. Go 3 miles on CR 17 to Stoneface Road and turn left. Continue 1.75 miles south on Stoneface Road to the entrance, on the left.

Saline County State Fish and Wildlife Area

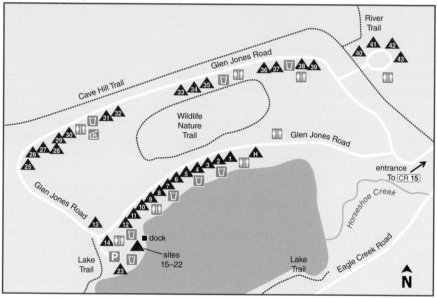

GETTING THERE

From US 45 in Harrisburg, drive east 9.5 miles on IL 13 to IL 142 at Equality. Turn right. Go 1 mile, then turn right at the brown park sign onto Walnut Street/CR 7. Follow the signs 4.5 miles to the left turn onto CR 15, then drive 0.5 mile to the park entrance, on the left.

GPS COORDINATES: N37° 41.493'   W88° 22.658'

45

Sam Dale Lake State Fish and Wildlife Area

Beauty ★★★★ Privacy ★★★★ Spaciousness ★★★★ Quiet ★★★★ Security ★★★★★ Cleanliness ★★★★★

It's well worth the walk to the scenic sites near the water's edge.

Sassafras Point Campground at Sam Dale Lake State Fish and Wildlife Area ranks very high on my list of near-perfect tent spots in a state park. It's completely separate from the RV campgrounds—it's on the opposite side of the lake, in fact. And it's scenic, being out on a point, meaning there's water on three sides. Its 21 walk-in sites are spread out, not in a line, with most just far enough from parking to attract only those who are passionate about privacy. Throw in a friendly little restaurant with a Sunday breakfast buffet, and you have an ideal place for a relaxed weekend getaway.

As you enter the park, go about 1.25 miles, heading past several roads to the right and the park office to the left, and turn right at the sign for Sassafras Point. There's a single parking lot and 21 amply shaded walk-in sites. Some sites are close to one another, but this campground is barely half full on a typical nonholiday weekend, so you shouldn't have to camp too near anyone else. You can go ahead and set up, then register with the campground host in Hickory Hollow (if available), or park staff will come by later to register you.

Most of these are great sites. Only 4 and 5 are too small; 7, 8, and 9 are in a line, so people camping farther down the point might walk through your camp. If you don't want to carry your gear far, sites 1 and 20 are right by the road—pull to the side,

Perfect campsite on Sam Dale Lake at Sassafras Point

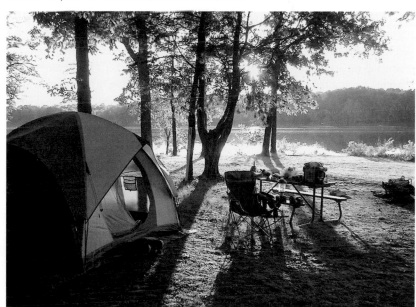

KEY INFORMATION

LOCATION: 620 CR 1910 North, Johnsonville, IL 62850

CONTACT: 618-835-2292, bit.ly/SamDaleIL

OPERATED BY: IDNR

OPEN: Year-round

SITES: Class B/E: 66 electric sites; Class C: 21 walk-in sites; group campground

EACH SITE HAS: Picnic table, ground grill; electricity in Class B/E only

WHEELCHAIR ACCESS: Restrooms and at least one accessible tent site

ASSIGNMENT: First come, first served; 12 sites reservable in Lakeview Campground

REGISTRATION: Set up first, then park staff will come by or go to the campground host at Hickory Hollow

AMENITIES: Water spigots, vault toilets

PARKING: At site; in lot (walk-in sites)

FEE: Class B/E: $18/night; Class C: $6/night

ELEVATION: 489'

RESTRICTIONS:

PETS: On leash only

QUIET HOURS: 10 p.m.–7 a.m.

FIRES: In fire rings only

ALCOHOL: Permitted

VEHICLES: 2 per site

OTHER: 14-day limit; 1 RV and 1 tent, or 2 tents per site; 4 adults or 1 family per site

unload, and then park. The only downside is being right next to everyone coming in and out. A bit farther out and well shaded are sites 3 and 21, both great choices. Sites 10, 13, and 17 are excellent, and 12, 14, and 15, which are closest to the water's edge, are nearly perfect. Site 12, the farthest, is well worth the 275-foot walk. It is close to 11, but if you get 12, you can hope that no other camping isolationist will take 11. On the water's edge is a bench, where at night I watched the sun go down over the lake, and in the morning sipped coffee while great blue herons swooped down from the trees to fish in the shallows.

Another nice option for privacy is the group campground, to the right as you enter the park. It's labeled "youth group" on the map but is available for any group, adults, or just a family, ranging from a handful to 50. It's not quite as attractive as Sassafras Point but is on the lake and has tables, grills, toilets, and water. You have to pay for a minimum of 10 people ($4 per adult), no matter how small your group is, but that might be well worth it if you want a place all to yourselves. It can be reserved, or you can register on arrival at the park office, if it's not already taken.

If you absolutely must have electricity, there are two Class B campgrounds on the other side of the lake. Hickory Hollow is the better choice, offering 33 wooded sites in a single loop. Of these, the sites at the outside back of the loop (11, 13, 14, and 15) seem less crunched together. Lakeview is the other campground. At the end of the road, it seems to be the busiest. All the Class B campsites are reservable online for $5 at reserveamerica.com.

On the road next to Sassafras Point you'll find the Middle of Nowhere—that's the name of the park's concession. They're open May 1–September 30, daily, 8 a.m.–7 p.m., and you can pick up ice, firewood, bait, and limited camping and fishing supplies. If you're tired of campfire cooking, the little restaurant offers a decent selection of sandwiches, salads, homemade pie, and nightly specials. As you pack up to leave on a Sunday, take advantage of their breakfast buffet. Call them at 618-835-2293 for more information.

Sam Dale Lake State Fish and Wildlife Area

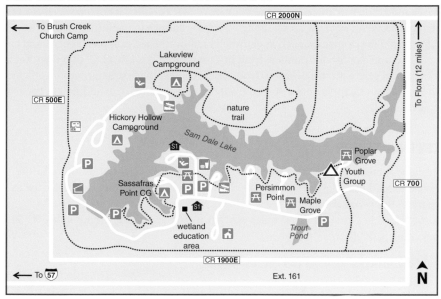

Sassafras Point Tent Campground

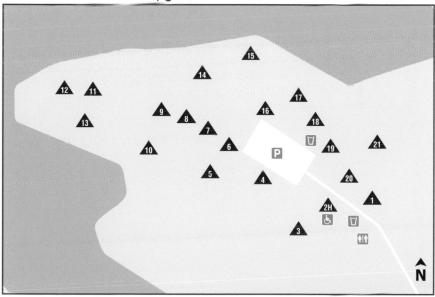

Anglers will enjoy fishing 194-acre Sam Dale Lake, whether by boat or along the shore-line from one of the picnic or camping areas. There is a boat launch next to Lakeview Campground, but you'll need to bring your own boat (under 10 horsepower); at present, the concession does not rent boats, though that may change in the future. In addition to the usual central Illinois species, such as catfish, largemouth bass, crappie, bluegill, and even a few muskie, you can fish for rainbow trout in Trout Pond: it is one of 55 sites that the IDNR stocks twice a year with this delicacy. Trout season opens the first Saturday in April and the third Saturday in October, and a special trout stamp is necessary in addition to the regular Illinois fishing license.

GETTING THERE

From Salem, take I-57 south to Exit 109. Go east on IL 161 about 22 miles to the large brown sign on the left for Sam Dale Lake. Turn left onto CR 700 East and drive 0.8 mile to the park entrance, on the left.

From IL 45 in Cisne, drive 7.2 miles west on IL 161 and make a right onto CR 700 East to reach the park entrance, on the left.

GPS COORDINATES: N38° 32.198' W88° 33.927'

46

Stephen A. Forbes State Recreation Area

Beauty ★★★★ Privacy ★★★★ Spaciousness ★★★ Quiet ★★★★ Security ★★★★★ Cleanliness ★★★★★

Don't miss the excellent sandy beach at Rocky Point.

The Stephen A. Forbes State Recreation Area offers tent camping with some luxury and plenty of convenient recreation for families. The separate walk-in tent area gets you away from the busy main campground, but nearby you still have showers, swimming, boating, a restaurant, and even a small store. It doesn't hurt that the park's 585-acre lake is beautiful, with 18 miles of timbered shoreline and more than 1,100 acres of surrounding forest to explore if you want more nature and fewer people.

Whether you enter Forbes from the east or west, turn left and follow the main road around the lake to the northwest and the Oak Ridge Campground. Chances are good that most if not all of the 115 sites here will be occupied by RVs on any weekend. Continue straight south through the campground, passing the shower house, playground, and pavilion, to reach the small parking lot for walk-in tent campers. There are only 10 sites here, spaced along a couple of short trails that head into the woods. This part of the campground is quieter and not nearly as busy. You might have it all to yourself midweek, and on nonholiday weekends usually no more than half the sites will be occupied.

You can park next to the closest sites, and the farthest is an easy walk of about 500 feet. You couldn't really call them isolated—the woods aren't dense, and there's not a lot of

Summer fun at the beach at Rocky Point

photo by Amy Fichter

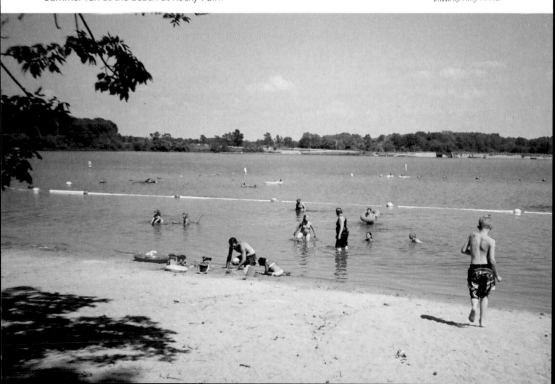

KEY INFORMATION

LOCATION: 6924 Omega Road, Kinmundy, IL 62854

CONTACT: 618-547-3381, bit.ly/SForbesIL

OPERATED BY: IDNR

OPEN: Year-round

SITES: Class A: 110 electric sites; Class B: 5 nonelectric sites; Class C: 10 walk-in sites; 1 cabin

EACH SITE HAS: Picnic table, ground grill

WHEELCHAIR ACCESS: Restrooms and at least one accessible electric site

ASSIGNMENT: First come, first served; reservations available online for 52 Class A sites and cabin

REGISTRATION: Register with the campground host if available; otherwise, set up and park staff will come by

AMENITIES: Water spigots, vault toilets, shower house (closed late Nov.–April 15)

PARKING: At site (Class A and B); in lot (Class C)

FEE: Class A: $20/night, $30/night holidays; Class B: $10/night; Class C: $8/night; cabin: $45/night ($5 reservation fee)

ELEVATION: 559'

RESTRICTIONS:

PETS: On leash only

QUIET HOURS: 10 p.m.–7 a.m.

FIRES: In fire rings only

ALCOHOL: Permitted

VEHICLES: 2 per site

OTHER: 14-day limit; 1 camping unit (RV or tent) or 2 smaller tents per site; 4 adults or 1 family of 6 per site

undergrowth separating the individual sites. Still, they're well shaded and about 75–100 feet from each other, which is much better than in the main campground. I prefer the farthest one, site 10, which offers the most space and the least chance that anyone will camp nearby. Sites 5–9 are all acceptable. Sites 3 and 4 are closer to each other, and 1 and 2 are too close to the parking lot. When I was there, site 1 was also muddy, even though none of the others were. If you want to stick close to your car, try site 6 instead. Once you've selected a site, register with the host at the campground entrance.

Continue down the trail about 500 feet past site 10 to reach the lake. Here you connect with the 2.5-mile Oak Ridge loop trail, which goes around the point and through the main campground. You can hike it either direction and, if you don't want to do the whole loop, return to your campsite via the campground road.

The lake is the star attraction at Forbes. There's an excellent 200-foot sandy beach at Rocky Point, on the southeastern corner, where you can swim all day for $2 per person. The beach is open daily from Memorial Day weekend to Labor Day, weather permitting, from sunrise to sunset. At the opposite corner of the lake, across the inlet from the campground, the marina rents motorized johnboats, pedal boats, and waterbikes. This is one of the few Illinois state park lakes with no horsepower limit, and about 1 mile of its length is open to waterskiing.

Anglers go for bluegill, crappie, and channel catfish on the lake, but it's especially known for largemouth bass. You can bank fish from the docks at the campgrounds, or from any of the picnic areas around the southern end of the lake. There are fish-cleaning stations at the campground entrance and at the Lakeview boat ramp on the east side.

After working up an appetite swimming, boating, fishing, or hiking, cross the inlet via the floating walkway to the restaurant and marina. This is one of the most attractive concession buildings I've seen at any Illinois park, with its landscaped waterfront, large dining room, and big picture windows overlooking the lake. At the time of writing, the park was in the process of looking for a new concessionaire for the restaurant, store, and marina, so details of menu and hours were uncertain. For more information, call the park offices.

If you're up for a challenging hike, about 20 miles north of Forbes is Wildcat Hollow, which seems like a piece of the Shawnee Forest transplanted north. The approximately 3.5-mile loop trail winds through upland forest, small canyons, and rocky streambeds—it starts easy, then gets rugged. You're sure to see wildlife—just don't go during deer-hunting season. Pick up a trail map at the Forbes office or online at bit.ly/WildcatHollowIL. To get there, head north to IL 37, turn right, then continue about 14 miles to Mason. Turn left on Main Street (CR 24), go 1.3 miles north, and turn right at the first intersection after I-57. Turn left on the gravel road and follow it to the parking lot.

For a different sort of outdoor challenge, check out the programs offered by nearby American Obstacle. You can experience ziplining over woods and water, kayaking, outdoor laser tag, and even team-building adventures for groups, all in a beautiful wooded setting on Kinmundy Lake. American Obstacle is located south of Kinmundy off IL 37. Go to americanobstacle.com or call 217-690-3367 for more information.

Stephen A. Forbes State Recreation Area: Walk-in Tent Area

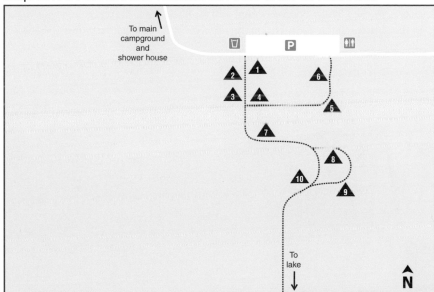

GETTING THERE

From I-57, take Exit 127 and head east on Kinoka Road 1.25 miles to Broom Road (CR 1475). Turn right and go 1.55 miles south to Williams Road (CR 1800). Turn left and drive 4.25 miles east to Omega Road (CR 27). Turn right and the park entrance is 1 mile straight ahead.

GPS COORDINATES: N38° 43.562'   W88° 46.826'

47

⛺ Trail of Tears State Forest

Beauty ★★★★ Privacy ★★★★★ Spaciousness ★★★★★ Quiet ★★★★★ Security ★★★★ Cleanliness ★★★★★

Camp in solitude at some of the most secluded yet accessible campsites in any state forest.

At Trail of Tears State Forest you won't find showers, electricity, playgrounds, swimming, fishing, boating, or even a pop machine. You will find more than 5,000 acres of beautiful, densely wooded, rugged hills—the easternmost outliers of the Ozarks, with long, narrow ridges and steep slopes that are more characteristic of neighboring Missouri than Illinois. Best of all, you will find 14 of the most secluded yet accessible campsites at any state park, where you can camp in solitude far from the nearest neighbor—assuming anyone else is even camping there.

Enter Trail of Tears on State Forest Road, which runs along an east–west valley. From there, two half-loop single-lane gravel roads climb into the hills to the north and south, follow a ridgetop, and descend again. Along each is sprinkled a handful of campsites, most of them excellent. Each has one or two tables, a ground grill, and a trashcan, and most have a pit toilet right at the site. (It may be an outhouse, but at least it's your own private outhouse!) I especially like the sturdy three-sided wooden Adirondack shelters found at four sites, built in the 1930s by the Civilian Conservation Corps. Each has a fireplace, and you can even camp in the shelter—pitch your tent on the floor, or simply hang a tarp over the entrance.

Register at the office in the historic white barn.

photo by J. M. Hagstrom

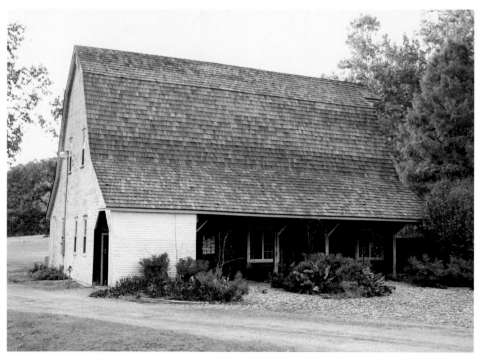

KEY INFORMATION

LOCATION: 3240 State Forest Road, Jonesboro IL 62952

CONTACT: 618-833-4910, bit.ly/TrailOfTearsIL

OPERATED BY: IDNR

OPEN: Year-round (all sites become hike-in only December 24–mid-May, when roads are closed)

SITES: Class C: 14; multiple hike-in sites; 1 group site

EACH SITE HAS: Table, ground grill, trash-can; 4 sites have 3-sided wooden shelter

WHEELCHAIR ACCESS: Not designated

ASSIGNMENT: First come, first served; reservations available online

REGISTRATION: Set up first, then self-register at the white barn

AMENITIES: Water spigot, vault toilets

PARKING: At campsite; along road (hike-in sites)

FEE: Class C: $8/night; hike-in sites: $6/night; $5 reservation fee

ELEVATION: 472'

RESTRICTIONS:

PETS: On leash only

QUIET HOURS: 10 p.m.–7 a.m.

FIRES: In fire rings only

ALCOHOL: Permitted

VEHICLES: 2 per site

North Forest Road is 4.2 miles long; follow it one-way counterclockwise, starting from its eastern junction with State Forest Road. Head uphill, and you'll first see site N1 (on the left), and then N2 (600 feet farther down the road), with a vault toilet between them. Another 0.25 mile brings you to N4 (on the left), then 1,000 feet later to N5; there's a toilet between these as well. All these sites are spacious and well shaded, but N2 is the largest and most attractive, perched on a ridge over a narrow wooded valley. Two adjacent sites, Y1 and Y2, are located at the northernmost point of the road. From here the road starts downhill, passing N6, N7, and N8, on the right, and finally N9, on the left at the bottom of the hill. N6 and N8 are beautiful—each has one of the large shelters, plenty of grassy space, and shade. N7 doesn't have a shelter and is a bit smaller, but it's still a great site. N9 is located in a large open clearing amid woods and doesn't have the view or shade of the sites farther uphill.

The other four campsites are along the 2.5 miles of South Forest Road, which also runs one-way, counterclockwise, beginning just across from the white barn housing the visitor center. Cross the concrete ford through the stream, head past the picnic area on the left, and climb the hill. From the T-intersection at the top of the hill, site S1 is on the right. You'll find one of the wooden shelters here, but it's smaller than the others, and the area in front of it is gravel. For a better option, turn left at the T-intersection and go 1.3 miles to site S2, my favorite spot on the south side; it has a larger shelter and plenty of space for multiple tents. Farther down the road are sites S3 and S4. Neither has a wooden shelter, but both are good—well shaded and spacious.

Youth or adult groups can camp by prior arrangement at the group area, which is off the south road. This area features a grill, a big fire ring surrounded by benches, and a neat outdoor amphitheater.

Wherever you settle, you'll need to get water at the spigot in front of the white barn on the main road through the park. That's also where you register at the self-registration station. Except during hunting season, which is just before and after Thanksgiving, you should always be able to find an open site on arrival. If you want to be sure to get a particular site, reservations are available in advance at reserveamerica.com for an additional $5. Camping is permitted year-round, but the north and south roads are closed from December 24–mid-May, so it's hike-in only then.

You can also backpack camp almost anywhere in the forest that's away from established campsites or picnic areas. Obtain a permit first from the visitor center (or check at the maintenance building behind the center) and be sure your vehicle doesn't block a road or fire lane.

Trail of Tears offers miles of hiking, equestrian, and fire trails, much of it fairly strenuous due to the hilly terrain. Be sure to bring a trail map (from the park brochure or online at bit.ly/TrailofTearsMap) and a compass or GPS unit because the trails are complex. A moderately difficult and pretty 2-mile trail loops through the Ozark Hills Nature Preserve on the south side. The trailhead is located between campsites S3 and S4.

While at Trail of Tears, don't miss the Pomona Natural Bridge, just 15 miles north. You can cross over and under this impressive 90-foot sandstone arch via a 0.3-mile loop trail. Take IL 127 north 10.8 miles to Pomona Road and turn left. Go 0.8 mile west to the three-way stop, turn right, and proceed 2.3 miles to the parking area.

Check the profiles of nearby Pine Hills and Turkey Bayou Campgrounds for many other sites to explore in the eastern Shawnee National Forest.

Trail of Tears State Forest

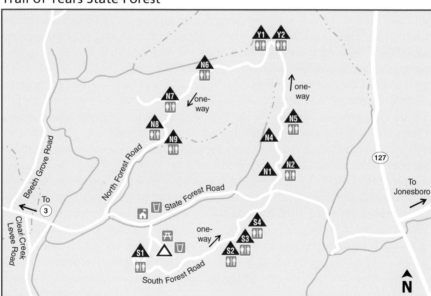

GETTING THERE

From US 51 and IL 146 at Anna, go 5 miles west on IL 146 to IL 127. Turn right and go 1.25 miles north to State Forest Road on the left. Turn left and drive 1.25 miles to the forest entrance.

GPS COORDINATES: N37° 29.289'   W89° 19.911'

48

⛺ Turkey Bayou Campground

Beauty ★★★ Privacy ★★★★★ Spaciousness ★★★ Quiet ★★★★★ Security ★★★★ Cleanliness ★★★★★

During the drier, cooler days of fall, Turkey Bayou is a quiet base camp for exploring the eastern Shawnee National Forest.

Turkey Bayou Campground is located between the Big Muddy River and Turkey Bayou, an abandoned oxbow lake of the Big Muddy. At 338 feet in elevation, this is just about as low as you can go in Illinois. It's surrounded by water and consequently can flood; in fact, from spring to mid-summer you're better off leaving it to the mosquitoes. During the drier, cooler days of fall, however, Turkey Bayou is a great place if you don't mind primitive sites. Outside of hunting season, chances are good you won't find many others there and can use it as a base for exploring some of the lesser-known sites of the eastern Shawnee Forest.

When I penned the first edition of this book, Turkey Bayou had only five poorly maintained sites, and was probably destined for closure by the U.S. Forest Service. Since then, however, a group of dedicated volunteers, the Friends of the Bayou, has contracted with the U.S. Forest Service to redevelop and maintain the campground. There are now 17 campsites, each with graveled parking, a fire ring, and a table. There are currently no water or toilet facilities.

The campground consists of a single loop, with 17 spacious sites, numbered counterclockwise. As you enter, stop at the information board on the right and sign the guest register—that lets the Friends of the Bayou and, more importantly, the U.S. Forest Service, know that maintaining this campground is worthwhile. There is no charge for camping, but you can place a donation in the receptacle. The sites on the right side of the loop have more tree cover, while

The Big Muddy River, from the boat dock near Turkey Bayou   *photo by Jeff Jinks*

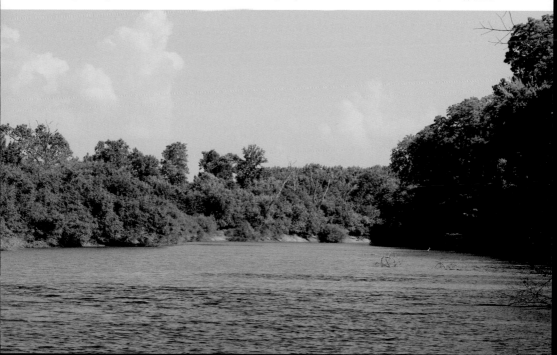

KEY INFORMATION

LOCATION: Oakwood Bottom Road, Pomona, IL 62975

OPERATED BY: U.S. Forest Service

CONTACT: Mississippi Bluffs Ranger District, 618-833-8576, bit.ly/TurkeyBayouIL

OPERATED BY: U.S. Forest Service

OPEN: Year-round

SITES: 17 tent sites

EACH SITE HAS: Picnic table, fire ring

WHEELCHAIR ACCESS: Not designated

ASSIGNMENT: First come, first served

REGISTRATION: No registration required

AMENITIES: None

PARKING: At site

FEE: Free, but donations accepted

ELEVATION: 338'

RESTRICTIONS:

PETS: On leash only

QUIET HOURS: 10 p.m.–6 a.m.

FIRES: In fire rings only

ALCOHOL: Permitted

VEHICLES: 2 per site

OTHER: 14-day limit; 8 campers per site

those on the left are closer to the river. If flooding is not a concern, I prefer those nearer the water. Bring a pole and you can fish right from your campsite. Bring a boat or canoe, and you can explore the river. Don't bring a swimsuit, though—the Big Muddy is aptly named and is home to venomous cottonmouth snakes.

This area is popular during hunting seasons, which in southern Illinois span from late November–late January. As you drive past the seasonal wetlands along Oakwood Bottoms Road on the way in, you can understand why this is prime waterfowl-hunting area. To view the wetlands from a dry 0.25-mile boardwalk trail, stop at Oakwood Bottoms Greentree Reservoir, 1 mile east of IL 3.

Across the Big Muddy River from the north of the campground you can actually look east into one of the neatest sites to explore in the Shawnee Forest: Little Grand Canyon. To get there, however, you have to get around the Big Muddy and approach from the east. Head 3.5 miles north of Oakwood Bottoms on IL 3 to Town Creek Road, where you'll see a sign for Little Grand Canyon. Turn right, go 5.6 miles to Maple Springs Road, and turn right again (Maple Springs will merge with Hickory Ridge Road). Go 6 miles to Little Grand Canyon Road, turn right, and proceed to the parking area. Three sides of the canyon are made up of steep sandstone bluffs, and its western end opens onto the Big Muddy River. A 3.6-mile loop trail descends into the canyon via steps cut into the rock then climbs back out, offering awesome views of the canyon and the Mississippi valley from the bluff tops. There are two trailheads by the parking lot—I suggest starting at the one by the restrooms and doing the loop clockwise. Be careful on the sandstone steps, which are steep and slippery when wet, and keep your eyes open for snakes—there are venomous ones around here. Don't descend into the canyon if there is a threat of heavy rain, as it can flood. For a good trail map, visit bit.ly /LittleGrandIL. Note that older maps and trail descriptions mention the Hickory Ridge lookout tower, but all that remains of it are a few concrete blocks by the parking lot.

Between the lowlands of Oakwood Bottoms and the Mississippi River to the west sits Fountain Bluff, a 4-mile-long sandstone hill that rises some 400 feet over the surrounding floodplain. At a distant point in geologic history, the bluff actually overlooked the western shore of the Mississippi River. Glacial ice forced the river westward to its present-day course, leaving Fountain Bluff a virtual island.

Today the hill is virtually unknown to tourists but offers some great views of the Mississippi, secluded canyons, and Mississipian Indian petroglyphs that have unfortunately been damaged by thoughtless visitors. To get to the bluff, head north on IL 3 from Oakwood Bottoms Road. Take the first left onto Happy Hollow Road to drive up the hill and explore from the top. To get to the canyons and petroglyphs, you have to approach from the northwest side. Continue north on IL 3 to Gorham Road, turn left, and go 1.2 miles into town to Second Street. Turn left, and head out of town toward the bluff. At about 1.1 miles, you'll see an isolated grove of trees on the right. Look for a trailhead to the left. Park off to the side; it's a short hike up to the petroglyphs. Just 0.2 mile farther down the road you'll see a parking area on the left. Here you'll find the entrance to a climbable little waterfall canyon leading to three small sandstone shelters. When I was there, someone had erected a couple of makeshift ladders to facilitate access, but one was starting to come apart, so use them with caution.

Turkey Bayou Campground

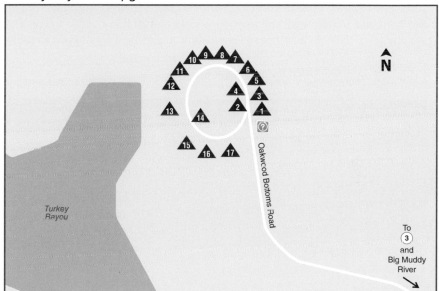

GETTING THERE

From Murphysboro, head west on IL 149 about 7 miles to IL 3. Turn left and head 5.9 miles south to Oakwood Bottoms Road. Turn left and go 4.5 miles to the campground.

From Jonesboro, head west about 8 miles on IL 146 to IL 3. Turn right and drive 17 miles north to Oakwood Bottoms Road. Turn right and it's 4.5 miles to the campground.

GPS COORDINATES: N37° 41.086'   W89° 24.630'

49

Washington County State Recreation Area

Beauty ★★★★ Privacy ★★★ Spaciousness ★★★★ Quiet ★★★★ Security ★★★★ Cleanliness ★★★★★

Washington County is a camping buffet—lots of great choices for tent campers.

Washington County State Recreation Area is kind of a camping buffet—you have a lot of choices. There are three different campgrounds, two especially for tent campers and one with walk-in sites. Throw in a 248-acre lake, showers, fishing, boating, and a convenient concession for supplies and snacks, and you have the recipe for a relaxing weekend.

Little Bear is the first campground you'll see as you enter the park—take the first right, and the next left. Little Bear consists of a single road with a loop at the end; stairs lead down to the lake and a fishing dock. It's a pretty, wooded, grassy area, with 20 unnumbered sites (numbered on my map for reference). Most sites offer plenty of room, and those on the right as you drive in (sites 1–7) are a bit farther apart. If you want to be close to the lake, sites 6 and 8 at the end are good—you can pop down the stairs to fish any time of the day or night. Site 12 has a small picnic pavilion next to it, which is great if it rains. The only sites I didn't like were 7, 10, and 11 (too small and sloping), and 19 and 20 (too close to the road). You won't see any gravel parking spots, but you're welcome to park on the grass next to your site.

Sunrise on the lake at Washington County

photo courtesy of Mike Kurtz Photography

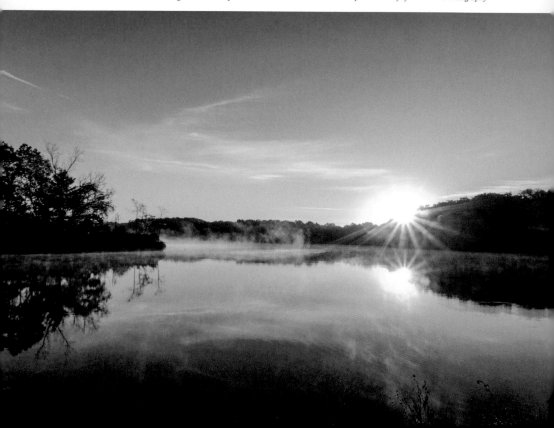

KEY INFORMATION

LOCATION: 18500 Conservation Drive, Nashville, IL 62263

CONTACT: 618-327-3137, bit.ly/WashCtyIL

OPERATED BY: IDNR

OPEN: Year-round

SITES: Class A: 51 electric sites; Class C: 52 nonelectric sites and 16 walk-in sites; 1 cabin

EACH SITE HAS: Picnic table, fire ring or ground grill; electricity in Class A only

WHEELCHAIR ACCESS: Restrooms and at least one accessible tent site

ASSIGNMENT: First come, first served; reservations available online (Class A and cabins only)

REGISTRATION: Register with the host or at the self-registration kiosk

AMENITIES: Water spigots, vault toilets, shower house (open April–October)

PARKING: At site (Class A and some Class C); in lot (walk-in)

FEE: Class A: $20/night, $30/night holidays; Class C: $8/night; $45/night for cabin; $5 reservation fee

ELEVATION: 499'

RESTRICTIONS:

PETS: On leash only

QUIET HOURS: 10 p.m.–7 a.m.

FIRES: In fire rings only

ALCOHOL: Permitted

VEHICLES: 2 per site

OTHER: 14-day limit; 1 RV and 1 tent, or 2 tents per site; 4 adults or 1 family per site

Note that youth groups frequent Little Bear. However, before you panic, thinking you might be overrun by a herd of Boy Scouts at midnight, know that groups have to make advance arrangements, and the sign at the entrance to the campground will indicate if it's been reserved for a group that day.

The next campground is Lonely Oaks—take the second right after the park entrance, then hang a left at the crossroads. Lonely Oaks has 32 unnumbered vehicle-access sites (numbered on my map for reference) along three prongs of a branching road, plus 5 walk-in sites. Site 6, on the right as you enter, is great, being well away from the road and shaded. Site 15, at the end of the middle fork, is in its own little wooded nook, and site 20 is on a flat, grassy area over the hill and next to the stairs leading down to the lake and fishing dock. Site 29, at the end of the left fork, offers a great view of the lake. Only the sites in the middle (18, 19, and 21–24) seem cramped and open. I camped at one of the walk-in sites at the end of the right fork and loved it. It's just a short walk from the parking lot (300 feet at most), and though there were others in the campground, I felt like I had the place to myself. As at Little Bear, you can park on the grass (except at the walk-in sites).

North of Lonely Oaks is the third campground, Shady Rest, with a single loop of 51 electric sites. The clean, excellent shower house is located at the entrance and open to all campers from April 1–October 31. Surprisingly, at the end of the loop there's also a parking lot and 11 walk-in tent sites. Five sites are right by the lot, but the other six are spread through the woods on a point overlooking the lake. For the best view, head to the one farthest out. Nearby are the park's two rental cabins, which have heat and air-conditioning, a table and chairs, beds for six, and a grill. This is a great combination if you have some family members who want a roof over their heads (like Mom and Dad), and others who want to tent camp nearby (like the kids). (Be sure to make cabin reservations well in advance at reserveamerica.com.)

Which campground to pick? Little Bear is smaller and more wooded, Lonely Oaks is more spread out, and the tent sites in Shady Rest are within walking distance of the showers. The electric sites at Shady Rest fill up most good weekends, but the tent areas are usually no more than half full outside of holidays. So browse the options, pick a site, and settle in. You can register with the campground host (if available) or at the self-registration kiosk near the showers.

The boat docks and park concession are south of Little Bear campground. There you can purchase ice, firewood, fishing tackle, bait, soft drinks, sandwiches, and snacks. If you'd like to explore the lake, you can rent kayaks or johnboats, with or without a motor. The concession is open April 1–October 31, daily, 7 a.m.–7 p.m.

Washington County Recreation Area has one official hiking trail: a 7-mile loop that circles the lake. Two-thirds of the loop follows the park road; the remaining wooded trail is rarely hiked and challenging to follow. The road portion is worth hiking or driving, though, as it passes through the woods on the eastern side of the lake, which most park visitors don't see. This is the best area for wildlife viewing, and the trees are beautiful in the fall.

GETTING THERE

From I-64, take Exit 50 and go south 7.5 miles on IL 127 through Nashville to Conservation Drive. Turn left and drive 1 mile to the park entrance.

GPS COORDINATES: N38° 16.818'   W89° 21.622'

Washington County State Recreation Area: Little Bear Campground

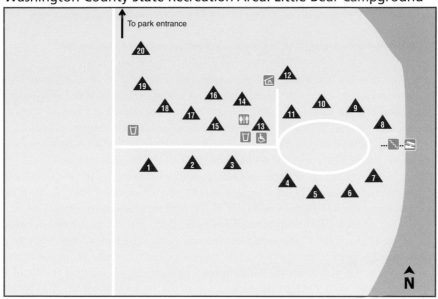

Washington County State Recreation Area: Lonely Oaks Campground

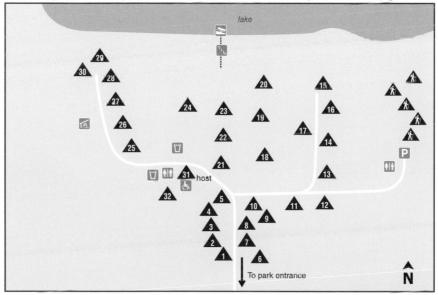

Wayne Fitzgerrell State Park

Beauty ★★★★ Privacy ★★★ Spaciousness ★★★ Quiet ★★★★ Security ★★★★ Cleanliness ★★★★

This ideal little tent campground lies amid a big outdoor recreational mecca.

If you search the web for "Rend Lake" in south-central Illinois, you'll find a resort, a golf course, a college, a marina, and several large and usually crowded RV campgrounds. It doesn't sound like the kind of place for a frugal tent camper hunting for more nature and fewer people. However, Wayne Fitzgerrell State Park offers an ideal little walk-in tent campground on a shaded point projecting into the lake. You'll rarely find solitude there, but you can camp in relative peace and still take advantage of all the lake has to offer.

Wayne Fitzgerrell is part of the huge outdoor mecca surrounding the 19,000-acre Rend Lake, managed jointly by the Illinois Department of Natural Resources, the U.S. Army Corps of Engineers, and the Rend Lake Conservancy. The park includes an enormous 248-site RV campground, but the walk-in tent area is all by itself to the north. In fact, it's far enough away from the main campground and resort that no one comes through except tent campers, and close enough that you can drive to all the amenities and recreational options available.

As you enter the park from the south, drive 3 miles north to just past the Rend Lake Resort. Turn right, go 0.5 mile, then make a left at the sign for tent camping. This road dead-ends at the loop, where you can park and walk to any of the 17 tent sites spread around the grassy point. In the middle of the loop you'll find the single water spigot, and the vault toilets to one side. Each site has a table and a ground grill.

Fall foliage adorns one of the many inlets on Rend Lake.   *photo by David Lauchner*

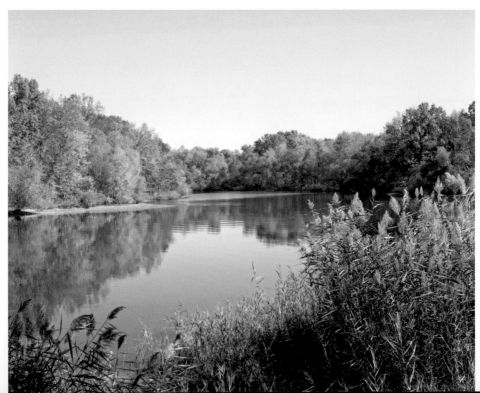

KEY INFORMATION

LOCATION: 11094 Ranger Road, Whittington, IL 62897

CONTACT: 618-629-2320, bit.ly/WFitzIL

OPERATED BY: IDNR

OPEN: Year-round (Class A); April 1–October 1 (Class C)

SITES: Class A: 248 electric sites; Class C: 17 walk-in tent sites

EACH SITE HAS: Electricity in Class A only; picnic table, ground grill

WHEELCHAIR ACCESS: Restrooms and at least one accessible electric site

ASSIGNMENT: First come, first served; reservations available online (33 Class A sites only)

REGISTRATION: Set up first, then register with the host in the Class A campground, otherwise with office staff

AMENITIES: Water spigots, vault toilets, showers

PARKING: At site (Class A); in lot (Class C)

FEE: Class A: $20/night, $30/night holidays; Class C: $8/night

ELEVATION: 417'

RESTRICTIONS:

PETS: On leash only

QUIET HOURS: 10 p.m.–7 a.m.

FIRES: In fire rings only

ALCOHOL: Permitted

VEHICLES: 2 per site

OTHER: 14-day limit; 1 RV and 1 tent, or 2 tents per site; 4 adults or 1 family per site

---

Most of the sites are well shaded and fairly far apart. Since this little campground may be busy on weekends, I suggest heading for the sites farthest out, so other campers won't be walking through or around your site to get to theirs. If you don't want to carry your gear far, try site 1, 2, or 3 to the east—they're far enough from the lot to give you some privacy, and there are no other sites behind them. However, I highly recommend heading away from the lot to the end of the point. Sites 6, 7, 8, 14, and 15 are closest to the lakeshore and offer beautiful views—you can watch the sun set to the west. Sites 14 and 15 are sunny; 6, 7, and 8 are more shaded. Just set up and then go register with a campground host in the Class A campground, or at the park office if no host is on duty. (If neither option is available, staff will come by the campground to register you.) Note that all campers can use the excellent shower facilities in the main campground.

If your easily bored kids (or you) prefer lots of activity to just sitting around the campsite, the Rend Lake area offers so much that you could all be exhausted by nightfall. Fishing, boating, and hunting are, of course, popular, but you can also enjoy swimming, hiking, mountain biking, horseback riding, golfing, disc golfing, and trap-shooting, or else visiting a winery, museums, and shops. Since the lake is large and the facilities spread out, scope out the options online in advance at bit.ly/USACE-RendLake or enjoyrend.com.

A good place to start at Rend Lake is the visitor center at the south end, on the west side of the dam. There you'll find not only current information but also interactive exhibits on the area, a live working beehive and pollinator garden, a 250-gallon aquarium featuring Rend Lake species, and terrariums of live snakes, turtles, and other area reptiles. Naturalists regularly lead free educational programs; check the events tab on their Facebook page for a schedule (facebook.com/rendlakeusace). The center is open daily from April–October, Monday–Friday, 8 a.m.–4 p.m.; and Saturday–Sunday, 9 a.m.–5 p.m. (closed on weekends November–March). From Wayne Fitzgerrell, go south through the park to IL 154, turn right, and continue across the lake to Rend City Road. Turn left, head south about 6 miles to reach Rend Lake Dam Road, and turn left again.

Swimming is available at the spacious South Sandusky beach on the west side of the lake, managed by the U.S. Army Corps of Engineers. (The North Marcum beach, which you may see mentioned in older brochures, is no longer a designated swimming area.) Visiting the beach costs $5 per car per day. You can take advantage of the hot showers and changing facilities there too. To reach it from the campground, cross the lake on IL 154 and head south on Rend City Road for about 3.25 miles to the South Sandusky entrance.

Other recreation options in the area include the 18-hole disc golf course at the North Sandusky Recreation Area, a 27-hole golf course at the Seasons Resort, 9 miles of equestrian trails, and some 20 miles of bike trail around the lake in three disconnected sections. The Rend Lake Marina, on the west side of the lake, rents motorized pontoon boats and fishing boats by the day. The Rend Lake Resort in Wayne Fitzgerrell State Park was closed at the time of publication, with the IDNR looking for a new concessionaire to manage it.

Wayne Fitzgerrell State Park: Walk-in Tent Campground

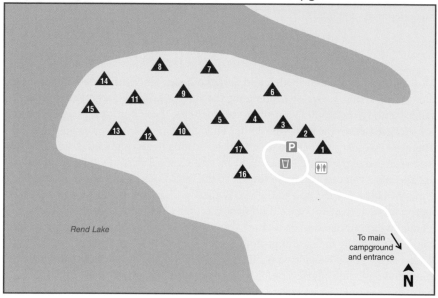

GETTING THERE

From I-57, take Exit 77 to IL 154 and head west 2 miles to the park entrance, on the right.

GPS COORDINATES: N38° 05.375'   W88° 56.869'

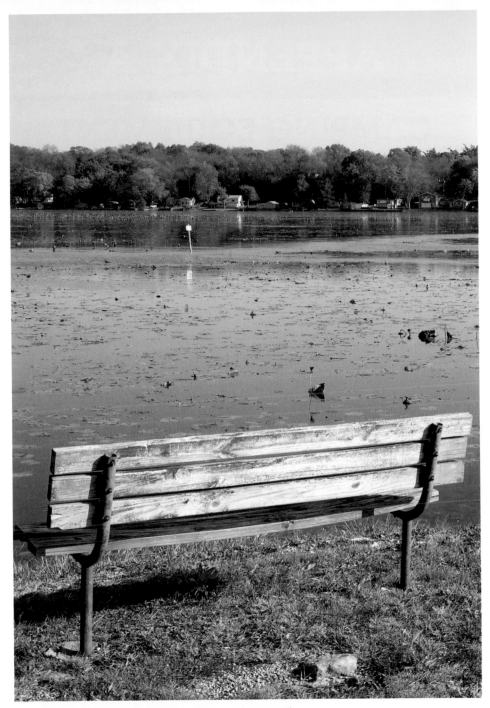

View of shallow Spring Lake from the causeway (see page 98)

APPENDIX A

CAMPING EQUIPMENT CHECKLIST

COOKING UTENSILS
Aluminum foil
Bottle opener
Can opener
Corkscrew
Cups (plastic or tin)
Dish soap (biodegradable), sponge, and towel
Flatware
Frying pan
Fuel for stove
Matches in waterproof container
Plates
Pocketknife
Pot with lid
Salt, pepper, spices, sugar, cooking oil, and maple syrup in spill-proof containers
Spatula
Stove
Wooden spoon

FIRST AID KIT
Antibiotic cream
Band-Aids
Diphenhydramine (Benadryl)
Gauze pads
Ibuprofen or acetaminophen
Insect repellent
Lip balm
Moleskin
Snakebite kit
Sunscreen
Tape, waterproof adhesive

SLEEPING GEAR
Pillow
Sleeping bag
Sleeping pad (inflatable or insulated)
Tent with ground tarp and rainfly

MISCELLANEOUS
Bath soap (biodegradable), washcloth, and towel
Camp chair
Candles
Cooler
Deck of cards
Duct tape
Fire starter
Flashlight or headlamp with fresh batteries
Foul-weather clothing
Paper towels
Plastic zip-top bags
Sunglasses
Toilet paper
Water bottle
Wool or fleece blanket

OPTIONAL
Barbecue grill
Binoculars
Field guides
Fishing rod and tackle
Hatchet
Kayak and related paddling gear
Lantern
Maps (road, topographic, trails, etc.)
Mountain bike and related riding gear

APPENDIX B

SOURCES OF INFORMATION

The following books and websites have been useful and enhanced my travels around Illinois.

BOOKS

Henry, Steve. *60 Hikes Within 60 Miles: St. Louis.* 3rd edition. Birmingham, Alabama: Menasha Ridge Press, 2010.

Villaire, Ted. *60 Hikes Within 60 Miles: Chicago: Including Wisconsin and Northwest Indiana.* 3rd edition. Birmingham, Alabama: Menasha Ridge Press, 2012.
Titles in the *60 Hikes Within 60 Miles* series contain the most detailed trail descriptions and maps you'll find anywhere. The St. Louis guide includes four hiking venues in Illinois.

Jeffords, Michael and Susan Post. *Exploring Nature in Illinois: A Field Guide to the Prairie State.* Champaign, Illinois: University of Illinois Press, 2014.
Vivid photographs and descriptions of the flora, fauna, and ecosystems of 50 parks and preserves around the state, including several in this book

Johnsen, David. *Biking Illinois.* Trails Media Group, 2006.
Detailed maps and trail descriptions covering the state

Post, Susan L. *Hiking Illinois.* 2nd edition. Champaign, Illinois: Human Kinetics, 2009.
This is my favorite hiking guide for the state as a whole, with detailed descriptions of 107 day hikes, including many around campgrounds I've included.

Rails-to-Trails Conservancy. *Rail-Trails Illinois, Indiana, and Ohio.* Birmingham, Alabama: Wilderness Press, 2017.
Excellent, detailed descriptions of biking trails built from former rail lines, including 27 in Illinois.

Svob, Mike. *Paddling Illinois: 64 Great Trips by Canoe and Kayak.* Madison, Wisconsin: Trails Books, 2007.
Some of the information on outfitters is outdated, but overall the descriptions of waterways and access points are detailed.

Ulner, Eric. *Vertical Heartland: A Rock Climber's Guide to Southern Illinois.* 3rd edition. Buncombe, Illinois: Vertical Heartland, 2005.
This is the definitive guide to the subject, covering not only where to climb but also specific routes, ratings, and recommendations. Order from verticalheartland.com.

Wiggers, Raymond. *Geology Underfoot in Illinois.* Missoula, Montana: Mountain Press, 1997. Engaging and entertaining, this volume reads like a travel guidebook, presenting the geology of selected sites around the state and explaining why the hills, valleys, rivers, and canyons look the way they do.

Friends of the Shawnee National Forest. *Equestrian and Hiking Trail Maps.* 2017.
These are the most up-to-date, detailed maps of the trails and sites in the Shawnee National Forest. One covers the eastern half, the other the western. They're printed on water-resistant paper, and 25% of the purchase price supports trail improvements. Order from shawneefriends.org.

WEBSITES

I FISH ILLINOIS: ifishillinois.org
The state's official fishing website. You'll find helpful information under "Places to Fish" and "Family Fishing Hotspots," and the weekly fishing reports on specific waterways will tell you what's biting and on what.

ILLINOIS HISTORIC SITES: www2.illinois.gov/dnrhistoric
Official gateway to all state historic sites

ILLINOIS STATE PARKS: www.dnr.illinois.gov/Parks
Illinois Department of Natural Resources' gateway to all state parks and other recreation areas

SHAWNEE NATIONAL FOREST: www.fs.usda.gov/shawnee
Home page of the Shawnee, which includes links to the most recent information about closings, restrictions, and changes. Click on the "Recreation" link for a helpful overview of all trails and recreational venues throughout the forest.

INDEX

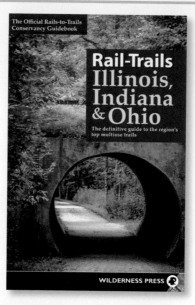
 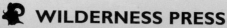

John Schirle was raised in central Illinois and has been back in his home state since 1993. During his college days, he developed a love for getting away in the outdoors—camping, hiking, canoeing, and, more recently, caving. As a result, he has spent countless hours scouring the region for the ever-elusive ideal tent-camping getaway. His personal goal for some years has been to visit every single state park in Illinois (he hasn't yet achieved this goal, but he's a lot closer now!). Over the years he has been a Bible translator in central Africa, a college professor, and a camp program director, and he is currently a children's librarian in his hometown of Decatur, Illinois.

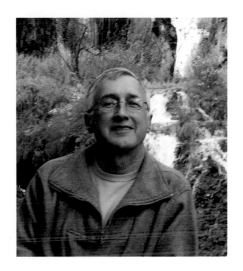

DEAR CUSTOMERS AND FRIENDS,

SUPPORTING YOUR INTEREST IN OUTDOOR ADVENTURE, travel, and an active lifestyle is central to our operations, from the authors we choose to the locations we detail to the way we design our books. Menasha Ridge Press was incorporated in 1982 by a group of veteran outdoorsmen and professional outfitters. For many years now, we've specialized in creating books that benefit the outdoors enthusiast.

Almost immediately, Menasha Ridge Press earned a reputation for revolutionizing outdoors- and travel-guidebook publishing. For such activities as canoeing, kayaking, hiking, backpacking, and mountain biking, we established new standards of quality that transformed the whole genre, resulting in outdoor-recreation guides of great sophistication and solid content. Menasha Ridge Press continues to be outdoor publishing's greatest innovator.

The folks at Menasha Ridge Press are as at home on a whitewater river or mountain trail as they are editing a manuscript. The books we build for you are the best they can be, because we're responding to your needs. Plus, we use and depend on them ourselves.

We look forward to seeing you on the river or the trail. If you'd like to contact us directly, visit us at menasharidge.com. We thank you for your interest in our books and the natural world around us all.

SAFE TRAVELS,

Bob Sehlinger

BOB SEHLINGER
PUBLISHER